"A game-changer for the healthcare industry…"

PHYSICIAN LEADERSHIP

THE Rx for HEALTHCARE TRANSFORMATION

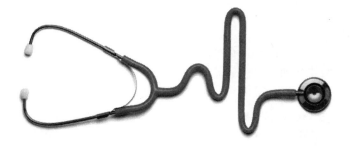

MoKasti

The Physician Leadership Institute

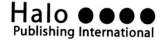

Halo ●●●●
Publishing International

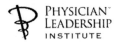

PHYSICIAN
LEADERSHIP
INSTITUTE

ISBN: 978-1-61244-216-7
Library of Congress Control Number: 2015900671

Printed in the United States of America

Halo ●●●● Published by Halo Publishing International
Publishing International 1100 NW Loop 410
Suite 700 - 176
San Antonio, Texas 78213
Toll Free 1-877-705-9647
Website: www.halopublishing.com
E-mail: contact@halopublishing.com

TABLE of CONTENTS

Introduction: What Must Be Done

THE SYMPTOMS

1. Industry Symptoms
2. Organizational Symptoms
3. Individual Symptoms

Dx: DIAGNOSIS

4. Lack of Engagement & Alignment
5. Why Physician Leadership Matters
6. Why Do Physicians Shy Away From Leadership?
7. Questionnaire: Assess Your Organization

Rx: PRESCRIPTION

8. Defining Physician Leadership
9. The Physician Leadership Model
   - Leading with Purpose
   - Leading with Strategy
   - Leading Self
   - Leading People
   - Leading for Results
10. Why Do Physician Leadership Programs Fail?
11. The Journey: Identifying & Closing the Gap
12. Alignment & Outcomes
   - Case Study: The Iowa Clinic
   - Case Study: The Physician Leadership Institute of Ohio
   - Interviews: Perspectives on Physician Leadership

A CALL TO ACTION
13. Physician Leadership: Where to Start?

"Progress occurs when courageous, skillful leaders seize the opportunity to change things for the better."

~ **Harry S. Truman**

Introduction:
What Must Be Done

The U.S. faces a watershed moment.

We must decide as a nation whether our citizens will live their lives in good health at a reasonable cost. At almost 18% of GDP, our current healthcare cost structure is unsustainable. The media headlines are bursting with stories and misinformation, often to the detriment of the healthcare industry.

Are we up to the challenge?

A few enterprising leaders have already made the shift; they have committed their lives and their organizations to a path of transformational change (we'll meet some of these leaders later in the book). While these leaders come from different backgrounds and organizations, they share one belief: **healthcare transformation is only possible under leadership provided by the ones who are the lifeblood of healthcare -** *physicians.*

The paradox is that physicians who should be in the vanguard of this transformation are missing for a myriad of reasons and in danger of being relegated to the sidelines. The danger is that in the absence of physician leadership, healthcare transformation will fail to materialize or resemble at best a patchwork of temporary solutions driven by short-term thinking.

The situation is dire because an increasing number of physicians seek early retirement citing "burnout" while more retrench between private practices and hospitals. Job dissatisfaction is at an all-time high resulting in more than 20% of physicians moving to a different hospital within the third year of their hire.

When physicians disengage from their vocations, whether due to cynicism or burnout, the transformation becomes impossible to achieve. Healthcare lags distressingly behind every sector, from business to manufacturing, in succession planning and leadership development.

Making things worse, today's medical education still focuses too narrowly on one aim: clinical skills. Medical schools are still mostly focused on graduating generations of physicians taught to treat patients in face-to-face interactions but not to assume the critical leadership roles required in our turbulent age. The focus is on individual excellence, not on quality outcomes, service delivery or value. We inadvertently keep producing doctors from the old paradigm while the new health age cries out for new skill sets that include leadership, teamwork, collaboration and innovation.

The impetus for us to invent the Physician Leadership Institute inside the Medical School at the University of South Florida was to connect the dots between a medical education (often focused on clinical skills with less focus on collaboration and empathy) and teaching leadership qualities, organizational skills and business acumen.

We believe physician leadership is not a position or a title. Rather, it is a mindset. We immerse the clinical mind of the practitioner in intensive action-learning experiences focused on developing leadership qualities, providing actionable feedback, and most importantly, integrating real-world applications of these leadership skills to solve real problems.

Where there is strong physician leadership, healthcare organizations benefit. They become purveyors of value - exemplars of quality patient care and cost effectiveness. Now more than ever, our industry needs physician leaders to make this value transformation a reality across healthcare organizations all over the country.

Organizations that effectively develop their physician leaders have demonstrated better engagement, better alignment and better results in health outcomes, patient and employee satisfaction, and business performance.

According to a recent study in the UK, hospitals that engaged their physicians in management roles improved their performance in key areas by 50% compared to peers with a low rate of physician engagement.

Executives are beginning to understand that strong leadership by physicians will be a key factor in how care is delivered in the future. For example:

- Britt Berrett, President of Texas Health Presbyterian Hospital in Dallas, announced his organization is moving toward a model where 65% of its executive leadership will be clinicians.

- Patrick Cawley, MD, CEO of Medical University of South Carolina Medical Center in Charleston, said his organization has created a Clinical Leadership Council, designed to bring together physician leaders to look at the big picture of what is best for the organization as a whole.

- Steve Newton, West Region President for Baylor Scott & White in Grapevine, Texas, said his organization created a physician leadership program to develop the clinical leaders the system needs for future success.

- C. Edward Brown, CEO of The Iowa Clinic, recognizes how the physician leadership has strengthened their culture and improved their ability to adapt to change and make bold strategic moves because they have "physicians leading physicians" with courage.

Under the auspices of the Physician Leadership Institute, this book will explain the genesis of such a leadership vacuum, highlight the symptoms facing physicians and healthcare organizations across various dimensions, provide a solution through the **Physician Leadership Model**™ that defines, measures, analyzes, improves and verifies leadership evolution, and provide real-life case studies where investments in physician leadership have paid off handsomely.

The book is divided into three main sections:

THE SYMPTOMS
We examine the various symptoms of the problems facing healthcare in the U.S. From global industry performance benchmarks to organizational and individual symptoms, we highlight the causes for dysfunction and the barriers to change.

Dx: THE DIAGNOSIS
We explore why there is a lack of physician engagement and alignment, **why physician leadership matters**, why do physicians shy away from leadership, and why leadership development programs fail? We then offer a diagnostics to assess your organization.

Rx: THE PRESCRIPTION
The first step to improvement is by understanding where we want to go. By envisioning the future and identifying the gaps in our competencies and capabilities, we can understand what we need to accomplish. How to accomplish this task is a function of leadership. Our **Physician Leadership Model** demonstrates the necessary foundational competencies required, from organizational purpose and alignment to individual leadership capabilities. We also define physician leadership in its simplest form.

The actual transformation is an ongoing process of closing identified gaps—the Physician Leadership Transformation Journey. We examine how best to structure your physician engagement initiatives, from strategy to execution.

We also investigate what it takes to sustain a culture of physician leadership. We include two case studies and a series of interviews with physician leaders.

Finally, the very last section in the book is a call to action, which asks you to think on seven questions as a leader and as a physician. Answering these questions will help you understand what your organization must do.

In my experience, **when medicine meets leadership** everything changes: the **culture**, the **care**, the way we **collaborate**, and most importantly, **outcomes**.

Healthcare transformation is not about high tech, but also about high touch. We need physician leaders. We can transform healthcare by rallying physicians and healthcare leaders to the urgency of leadership and its impact on the transformation.

I would like to thank every physician and leader we had the privilege of working with on transforming their "self," teams and organizations. Special thanks to Dr. Steve Klasko for his leadership at USF Health, and to Edward Brown and Dr. Daniel Kollmorgen from The Iowa Clinic, Ed Lopez from CHI, Dr. Lennox Hoyte from USF Health, and Dr. Joe Cooper for their thoughtful insights. Thank you to everyone at the Physician Leadership Institute for the commitment, passion and dedication.

I would also like to thank my dear family – Rana, Adam and Jude- for their love, support, patience and encouragement.

Finally, thanks for picking up this book. I hope it will help you see that Physician Leadership makes all the difference.

Sincerely,

Mo Kasti
Founder,
The Physician Leadership Institute™
www.physicianleadership.org

"THE SYMPTOMS"

Industry Symptoms:
Where's the Value?

Hardly a day goes by without an article in the media about the dismal performance of the U.S. healthcare industry. The "facts" are examined and debated, even politicized, but in the end the reality is we can and must do better. Performance data for the U.S. healthcare industry allows us to see what's going on.

Here are a few examples of industry "symptoms" that reveal the current state:

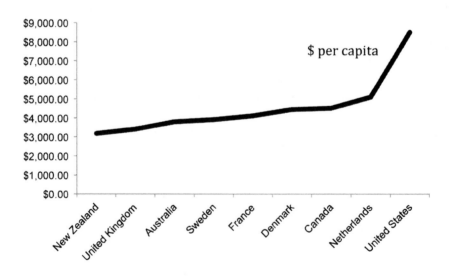

The U.S. spends *more* per–capita on healthcare than other industrialized countries.

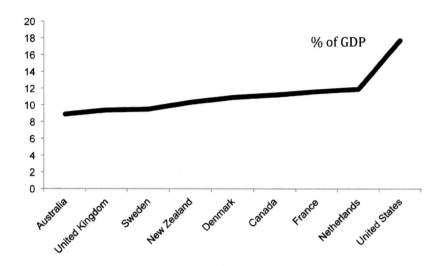

The U.S. also spends *more* as a percentage of GDP on healthcare than the other industrialized countries.

Overall the picture is rather bleak:

- The U.S. taxpayer subsidizes healthcare costs without always receiving any benefits

- Healthcare spending in the U.S. has grown much faster than the rest of the economy in recent decades

- Despite high spending, U.S. citizens don't go to the doctor very frequently

- Hospital stays in the U.S. aren't long, but they cost more than stays in other countries

- Commonly prescribed drugs are far more expensive in the U.S.

- Hospital visits for chronic conditions are significantly higher in the U.S.

- U.S. citizens don't enjoy longer lifespans than people in countries spending much less on healthcare

- Healthcare spending in the U.S. is projected to double in the next decade

(See: "Why U.S. Health Care Is Obscenely Expensive, In 12 Charts," *Huffington Post*, October 3, 2013)

The U.S. healthcare industry is also experiencing a seismic shift along several dimensions at the same time.

Market Place Consolidation
While industry consolidation has tremendous potential to improve patient care, it also risks driving up the cost. How this tension is resolved will determine whether health system changes ultimately benefit patients.

New Models of Care Delivery
The Patient Protection and Affordable Care Act (PPACA), commonly known as "Obamacare" or simply ACA, offers incentives to develop, test and evaluate new models of care and delivery systems. These changes will not be easy and will require physician leadership to meet the transformational challenges ahead.

Waste
It is estimated that wasted healthcare spending in the U.S. accounts for $765 billion annually. "Waste" is categorized as unnecessary services, excessive administrative costs, prices that are too high, fraud, inefficiently delivered services and missed prevention opportunities (*The Healthcare Imperative: Lowering Costs and Improving Outcomes*, Institute of Medicine, National Academy of Sciences, 2010).

Transparency and Competition

Now, for the first time, the Centers of Medicaid and Medicare Services (CMS) have released comprehensive data on the costs of the 100 most common inpatient procedures performed in 3,000 hospitals and medical centers across all 50 states.

At the Physician Leadership Institute, we went through the data on joint replacement surgeries without medical complications and co-morbidities (i.e. reasonably healthy patients who undergo knee or hip surgery for degenerative joint changes). The baby boomer generation entering their 6th decade is the quintessential demographic for such surgeries with an assurance of a good quality of life thereafter. No small wonder orthopedic surgery is the top earning specialty in hospitals and medical centers.

However, costs fluctuate wildly between states, intra state and even within hospitals located within a stone's throw from each other in the same city. In a southern state like Alabama, the average covered charges for joint replacements works out to $52,613. In California, three time zones away, the average was almost twice as much, at $90,000. Within Alabama, for example, Stringfellow Memorial Hospital at Anniston was the most expensive charging $141,035, while 106 miles to the northwest, Parkway Medical Ctr. in Decatur would set a patient back the least at $21,006. In Birmingham, the most populated state city, the six hospitals listed varied in price from $31,093 at St. Vincent's East to $89,408 at Trinity Medical Ctr. The difference was more than $60,000 within a few miles, or to put it in a different perspective, the cost of three such surgeries in Decatur.

This phenomenon is repeated in California with a $223,373 bill for a hip replacement at Monterey Park Hospital, Monterey but within the same county, Kaiser Foundation Hospital at Downey charges $32,358 or the difference of nine such procedures in Decatur, AL.

What about the University of California Medical System? Surely, their costs would be reasonable. At an average of over $95,000 they were anything but. Curiously, such costs remained impervious to socioeconomic conditions. In cash strapped Bakersfield-Modesto-Fresno, one of the country's poorest metros where almost one in four live below the poverty line, the cost for joint replacement averages at $87,000.

The Quest for Value

In his now classic article "What is the Value in Healthcare?" (*The New England Journal of Medicine*), business guru Michael Porter points out that in healthcare, the "stakeholders have myriad, often conflicting goals, including access to services, profitability, high quality, cost containment, safety, convenience, patient-centeredness, and satisfaction. Lack of clarity about goals has led to divergent approaches, gaming of the system, and slow progress in performance improvement."

According to Porter:

> *Achieving high value for patients must become the overarching goal of health care delivery, with value defined as the health outcomes achieved per dollar spent.*

Porter's formula is a unifying purpose for all stakeholders involved because value depends on outcomes and centers on the patient. But Porter goes further. Outcome measurement and costs should be measured separately – he emphasizes, because we actually know very little about cost from the perspective of examining the value delivered for patients. The problem according to Porter:

> *Understanding of cost in health care delivery suffers from two major problems. The first is a cost-aggregation problem. Today, health care organizations measure and accumulate costs for departments, physician specialties, discrete service areas, and line items (e.g. supplies or drugs). As with outcome*

measurement, this practice reflects the way that care delivery is currently organized and billed for. Today each unit or department is typically seen as separate revenue or cost center. Proper cost measurement is challenging because of the fragmentation of entities involved in care. Entities such as rehabilitation units and counseling units are all but ignored in cost analyses. Costs borne in outpatient settings, particularly within primary care practices are often not counted. Past efforts at cost reduction reflect the way costs are accumulated. The focus has been on incremental steps and quick fixes. Payers have haggled over reimbursement rates, which are not the true underlying costs.

Also, consider:

Past efforts at cost reduction reflect the way costs are accumulated. The focus has been on incremental steps and quick fixes. Payers have haggled over reimbursement rates, which are not the true underlying costs. There are efforts to raise the efficiency of individual interventions rather than examine whether there is the right group of interventions. Considering drugs as a separate cost, for example, only obscures the overall value of care and can lead to misplaced efforts to reduce pharmaceutical spending, rather than more holistic approaches to improving efficiency over the full cycle of care. The net result has been marginal savings at best and sometimes even higher costs.

There are no simple solutions. Porter tells us the full reimbursement for a total joint replacement in Germany or Sweden is approximately $8,500, including all physicians' and technical fees, and excluding only outpatient rehabilitation. The comparable figure for the United States is on the order of $30,000 or more. Why? Unfortunately, most physicians and provider organizations are not aware of the total cost of caring for a particular patient or group of patients over the full cycle of care.

In fact, businesses such as Home Depot and Walmart have selected four major providers across the U.S. where their employees may receive hip replacements. They determined these providers deliver the most value.

Why has this happened?

In an interview for this book, we asked Dr. Lennox Hoyte at the University of Southern Florida to share his perspectives. Dr. Hoyte is a board certified OB/GYN physician and fellowship-trained in Urogynecology and Female Pelvic Medicine and Reconstructive Surgery. He's one of the leading robotic prolapse surgeons in the world.

Here's Dr. Hoyte:

> *As our industry is challenged to improve accountability and outcomes, physicians are going to need to drive the change.*
>
> *For example, most doctors (myself included) do not know the costs of the treatment plans that we offer our patients. Many of us are disconnected from the business side of activities. I think that this is unacceptable. We need to gain a better understanding of the costs of the services that we offer to our patients; so that we can help to drive these costs down.*
>
> *Also, because of the increasingly interdisciplinary nature of patient care, doctors will be required to become more collaborative team players, skilled at initiating and managing change. That can't and won't happen without physician leadership.*

Organizational Symptoms

At the Physician Leadership Institute, we find most organizational challenges facing healthcare institutions fall under two broad categories:

(1) Strategic Confusion
    a. Transformation Anxiety
    b. Intensity and Accelerated Rate of Change
    c. Unclear Vision and Direction
    d. Value Based Care Transformation
    e. Shifting Risk
    f. Increased Competition
    g. Expanded Health Team
    h. Physician Employment
    i. Undefined Strategy for Physician Engagement

(2) Cultural Weakness
    a. Physician Turn Over and Retirement
    b. Lack of Loyalty to the Organization
    c. Lack of Effective Onboarding
    d. Variations in Practices and Outcomes
    e. Lack of a Quality Improvement Culture
    f. Lack of a Patient-Focused Care Culture
    g. Lack of Cost Accountability
    h. Very Limited Joint Outcomes Accountability
    i. Lack of Unity (Us vs. Them)
    j. Lack of Trust

We see a common set of challenges that keep recurring. It should come as no surprise that many of these challenges are directly related to **physician engagement** or rather, the lack of it.

Strategic Confusion

As we take a closer look at the challenges faced by many healthcare organizations, we can name the common "symptoms" and begin the diagnostic process. These symptoms fall under a category we call **strategic confusion**—that is, there is not a common understanding or shared vision for the strategy of the institution. Communications may or may not be plentiful, but clarity and unity of purpose are lacking.

Transformation Anxiety

Over the years, every industry has undergone a transformation from the Craft Age to the Industrial Age, and then to the Information Age. According to business guru Daniel Pink, we are going through yet another transformation now; this time from the Information Age to the Conceptual Age—an age that demands "empathy" and constant "innovation." Unlike other industries, healthcare has been slow to meet the change imperatives demanded by society. It is still going through its own transformation from the Craft Age (where every physician approaches his/her work as a Craft) to the Industrial Age, and finally with Health IT, to the Information Age.

Intensity and Accelerated Rate of Change

Compared to other industries, healthcare is going through a rapid pace of change that leads to a series of well-intentioned change initiatives that overwhelm both staff and physicians. The result? Change initiatives are viewed as just another "flavor of the month" and are not taken seriously by practitioners.

Unclear Vision and Direction

With the intensity and accelerated rate of change, senior administrators are struggling with dealing with many market factors showing up at the same time, such as increased competition, market consolidation, new model of care, physician alignment, patient centered care, bundled payment, ACO operational efficiency and effectiveness, thus sending mixed messages about vision and direction to front-line healthcare professionals struggling to meet the day-to-day performance requirements. Left unaddressed, this lack of clarity and direction leads to confusion, stress, burnouts and under-performance. There is a failure to "connect the dots."

Value-Based Care Transformation

Michael Porter's "value-based competition" is a positive-sum competition in which all system participants can benefit. When providers win by delivering superior care more efficiently, patients, employers and health plans also win. When health plans help patients and referring physicians make better choices, assist in coordination and reward excellent care, providers benefit. Just how will organizations manage this transformation?

Shifting Risk

Due to the fragmentation of the healthcare industry, trust and collaboration are not natural among the various stakeholders: government, health plans, payers, hospitals and physicians. As risk is being shifted among those participants, who are not yet clear on how the pie will be divided, table manners are lost.

Increased Competition

Locally and regionally, competition between healthcare providers will lead to a renewed focus on efficiency and process improvement. It is unclear who will lead the change or even what is required to make the transformation possible.

Expanded Health Team

The Patient Protection and Affordable Care Act (PPACA) authorizes states to establish community-based interdisciplinary or inter-professional teams to support primary care practices within a certain area. The "Health Teams" discussed in PPACA may include nurses, nurse practitioners, primary care physicians, medical specialists, pharmacists, nutritionists, dietitians, social workers and providers of alternative medicine. The "Health Team" is expected to support patient-centered medical homes, which are defined as models of care that include personal physicians, whole person orientation, coordinated and integrated care, and evidence-based medicine.

Physician Employment

As healthcare systems employ more and more physicians, there is a tendency for resentment amongst physicians who value their autonomy and do not like to be treated as "employees." This creates a barrier between individual priorities and organizational objectives—often exacerbated by a lack of trust.

Undefined Strategy for Physician Engagement

Physicians are the lifeblood of a healthcare organization and engaging them in leading such a transformation is very critical and essential. Many healthcare institutions worry about alignment, but few take the time to establish an end-to-end strategy, let alone an action plan for physician engagement.

The strategic challenges mentioned above are simply a list to demonstrate the depth and scope of change imperatives faced by the healthcare industry. We need engaged physician leaders if we are to achieve the transformation and the best medical outcomes for patients.

CHECKLIST: Ask yourself if you see the following symptoms.

- ☐ Misaligned goals between hospitals and physicians
- ☐ Anxiety about the future of healthcare
- ☐ Providers unaware of the financial implications of their actions on the system
- ☐ Confusion about the strategic direction of the organization
- ☐ Resistance to change and preserve the status quo
- ☐ Limited adoption of evidence based practices
- ☐ Lack of physician engagement in clinical transformation efforts, including patient experience
- ☐ Physicians limiting their involvement to clinical work

Cultural Weakness

We just highlighted the symptoms of the lack of strategic leadership hindering effective healthcare transformation. In the same manner, cultural aspects can prove to be serious stumbling blocks along the way to transformation. Here are a few cultural symptoms of weakness:

Physician Turn Over and Retirement

"Turnover in medical groups continues to climb along with the economy," says Lori Schutte, president of a healthcare recruiting firm in St. Louis, Missouri. [*Physician Turnover Rate Rises With Economy, Robert Lowes, Medscape Medical news, March 18, 2013*] When Cejka and the AMGA broke down physician turnover by group size, they found smaller groups had a faster revolving door. Practices with 3 to 50 physicians posted the highest turnover rate — 11% — in 2012. Similarly, the retirement rate among physicians aged 64 years topped out at 19% in this group category. In comparison, it was only 10.8% in groups of 151 to 500 physicians and 12.7% in those with more than 500.

Another finding: younger physician generations are not interested in getting involved and would rather spend time with family than in meetings. Succession problems are particularly pronounced in the healthcare sector given there are few formalized programs in medical school that stress leadership qualities. The leadership evolution also takes time and must go beyond self-help books and seminars.

Lack of Loyalty to the Organization

Physician retention failure and early retirement is becoming all too common. Fully 20% of physicians find new jobs within the third year of hiring. Again, aligning themselves to the organization and its values provides a huge challenge.

Lack of Effective Onboarding

Over the past years, physician turnover has accelerated alarmingly. Surveys show more than 20% of physicians change jobs within the second to third year of practice. Many others seek early retirement citing burnout and reimbursement challenges. Migration from private practices to hospitals has increased precipitously leading to increased competition. Unfortunately, few organizations have formalized on-boarding programs that cement commitment and improve retention.

Variations in Practices and Outcomes

Increasingly, providers use evidence-based research to drive treatment and outcomes with performance-based indices that measure improvement. Many still lag behind leading to significant variations nationally in treatment and prevention. Physician leadership is critical to engage their peers in meaningful clinical practice debates and accountability to reduce variations.

Lack of a Quality Improvement Culture

"A rising tide lifts all boats" was JFK's mantra for the economy, but it is equally applicable to healthcare where centers of excellence have significantly benefited from physicians pushing for improving quality from all levels of the organization. Unfortunately, this collective culture has yet to permeate widely, leading to frustratingly fluctuating levels of healthcare quality.

Lack of a Patient-Focused Care Culture

Healthcare organizations face increasing competition— empowered patients with access to better information, delivery models that stress performance metrics and quality of healthcare, and reimbursement depending on those outcomes.

Lack of Cost Accountability

As we mentioned earlier, the U.S. spends more dollars per patient on healthcare than any other country in the world (17.6% of its GDP on healthcare as compared to the OECD's average of 9.5%). Increasingly, the pressure to deliver healthcare with a cost-benchmark will drive massive changes in how work gets done. Unfortunately, our physicians are ill prepared for this change. Most have no idea what a procedure costs or what part they play in the total billing of a patient.

Very Limited Joint Outcomes Accountability

Institutional leaders can push for improvement in clinical outcomes (i.e. bringing down infection rates or falls) but this strategic vision should be channeled from Medical Executive Committee to service leaders in charge of their units and thereon to the front line physicians, making the desired outcome a collective responsibility. Getting everyone on the same page remains one of healthcare's foremost challenges and the primary reason why outcomes aren't achieved.

Blaming Each Other (Us vs. Them)

More and more reimbursements are being tied to perfomance metrics, which not only covers treatment and outcomes, but also, careful electronic documentation. The mantra is cost efficiency and minimizing wastage: exposing fault lines between front line physicians concerned about patient care and administrators concerned with bottom lines, leading to unproductive finger pointing.

Lack of Trust

Talking over one another rather than to each other has become the norm. Organizations do not emphasize emotionally intelligent leadership that relies on empathy and self-regulation in building bridges. Aligning oneself to the goals of the organization remains a huge challenge when doctors who take leadership roles are regarded as "sellouts" or labeled "gone to the dark side" while administrators are derided as "know-nothings."

These cultural aspects coupled with the temptation of executives and senior managers to drive change via top-down directives could backfire. The blowback is even more dysfunction, higher costs, higher turnover rates and predictably poorer performance.

CHECKLIST: Ask yourself if you see the following symptoms.

- ☐ High physician turn over
- ☐ Processes are clinician centric versus patient centric
- ☐ Variations in practices and outcomes
- ☐ *Us-Versus-Them* behaviors
- ☐ Win-lose versus win-win discussions and negotiations
- ☐ Lots of blame without engagement in problem solving
- ☐ Lack of cost accountability
- ☐ Physicians skeptical about the administrative agenda
- ☐ Hard to agree on evidence-based protocols citing "uniqueness" of practice or patient mix

Individual Symptoms

We've seen how cultural weaknesses and strategic confusion impact the healthcare transformation. Now let's turn to a third and vital challenge—the individual. Specifically, let's examine the **signs** that serve as warning flags. Here are some examples:

a. Lack Leadership Skills
b. Lack of Adaptability
c. Insufficient Physician Change Agents
d. Failure to Show Empathy
e. Relationships Based on Trust
f. Failing to Recognize Others
g. Stress and Burnout
h. Disruptive Behavior
i. The Language of Blame
j. Unhealthy Conflicts
k. Already a Leader

Lack of Leadership Skills
Healthcare, compared to other sectors, significantly lags behind in producing leaders. Current medical education and credentialing are devoid of leadership training and team-building, focusing more narrowly on clinical skills. The current system also disincentivizes physicians from active leadership roles. This is a key point. Let us recall hospitals where clinicians engage in management improved their performance by 50% as compared to hospitals with low clinician participation.

Lack of Adaptability
Charles Darwin once said, "It is not the strongest of the species that survives, nor the most intelligent that survives. It is the one that is most adaptable to change." Unfortunately,

physicians tend to be more analytical thinkers and part of the "expert culture" with less flexibility and creative qualities that could be vital to transformation.

Insufficient Physician Change Agents

A change agent is a catalyst who eschews bias that stagnate an organization and awakens dormant creative and collaborative qualities in others to achieve qualitative transformation.

Physicians have not been trained to be change agents with the necessary skills to assess, engage, influence, enlist and awaken the possibilities in others. A set of physician biases ranging from entrenched hierarchies, lack of trust and risk-averse behavior impede the development of such change agents.

Failure to Show Empathy

Successful leaders show what Daniel Goleman terms "emotional intelligence" and one of its aspects is self-regulation or the ability to break destructive habits and regulate disruptive emotions that govern adaptability. Research shows medical students show an alarming drop in empathy, a critical component of "emotional intelligence," between their first and third year of training. The "broken covenant" in healthcare further increases cynicism in physicians, sapping the motivation needed for patient-centric care, organizational commitment and leadership qualities.

Building Relationships

Physicians tend to focus their energy and time on clinical problem solving and dealing with the increased demands for documentation and performance; leaving less time for building relationships with peers, clinical team and administrative team. These relationships are very important in building trust and leading to higher retention rates.

Failing to Recognize Others

Another fall-out from the expert culture vs. collaborative culture is the inability of physicians to appreciate the role of others in healthcare success and build collaborative teams.

Stress and Burnout

Healthcare's broken covenant, where physicians feel the brunt of governmental regulations, income limitations and loss of stature, has led to the all too common phenomenon of burnout. Many cite this is due to the exorbitant amounts of money needed to set up practice, pay hundreds of thousands of dollars in liability, litigious nature and failing reimbursement rates. There has been an exodus of physicians into the safer havens of hospitals with private practices falling to less than 30% from 50% a decade ago.

Disruptive Behavior

Emotionally intelligent individuals are self-aware, regulate their own behavior, show empathy, motivation and have very good social skills. These have been shown as hallmarks of good leadership. At the other end of the spectrum are those who play victim and the blame game, show disinterest, do the minimum and are happy with the status quo, resentful of success, inflexible and reactive.

The Language of Blame

Do physicians walk into a meeting blaming everyone else about an issue or do they come in with the following statement: *"We own this issue and let's identify the solution together?"* The blame game is a symptom of the lack of alignment between the physician and the organization. Effective leadership results in a sense of collective responsibility.

Peter Drucker stressed the importance of self-report and feedback analysis where expected results are matched to actual results and the reason for shortfall becomes a collaborative process. Highly motivated leaders never complain when things don't go their way. Instead they re-channel their energies to engage in identification of the solutions. They show a passion for work that goes beyond their own personal gains. Goals are pursued with energy and persistence. Their commitment inspires others to do the same.

Unhealthy Conflicts

In many conflict style assessments, physicians tend to fall into one of two styles: they either avoid or confront conflict. Physicians in their medical training and credentialing are given no exposure to conflict resolution, which results in either avoidance behavior or a confrontational style that stymies team building and organizational alignment. Highly effective leaders are extremely self-aware, self-disciplined and show the empathy to deal with conflicts effectively.

"Already a Leader"

I'm already a leader—alright? What are you bothering me for? I can tell you right now what the clinic needs to do; you just need to listen to me. I don't have time for this stuff. These were the words of Dr. Kollmorgen of The Iowa Clinic **before** attending the Physician Leadership Institute.

His view is common. For physicians, the intrinsic feeling is the organizations they work for should align themselves to *their* expertise. However, transforming the healthcare paradigm requires many different building blocks: leadership skills, patient centricity, a collaborative culture and business acumen that are unfortunately absent from the clinical heavy curricula established in medical schools and a credentialing process failing to test them in these aspects.

The result is generations of physicians trapped; blocked off from active leadership roles because of functional illiteracy in the executive and collaborative cultures, and worse, many develop a contempt that precludes them from participation even when such opportunities arise. Fortunately, change is possible.

After attending the Physician Leadership Institute, Dr. Kollmorgen's views changed. *I do have some new perspectives. I now admit that listening is the #1 leadership skill... Soft stuff is my weak spot... Life is about relationships... I want to live in an enlightened state, not just someone who has the wisdom, but someone who has a big picture view.*

Dr. Kollmorgen is now a leading proponent of physician leadership and we'll hear more from him later in the book.

CHECKLIST: Ask yourself if you see the following symptoms.

- ☐ Interactions focused on tasks with little or no relationship building
- ☐ Use of the language of blame instead of ownership
- ☐ Empathy erodes as physicians suffer burnout and organizational drift
- ☐ Physicians shying away from leadership development – "Already a Leader" perception
- ☐ Not enough physician change agents engaged and influencing their peers
- ☐ Unproductive communication and meetings
- ☐ Increased physician stress and burnout
- ☐ Unhealthy conflicts and increased disruptive behaviors

Dx: THE DIAGNOSIS

Engagement & Alignment

In 2005, a survey of **physician engagement** was conducted by the **Gallup** organization. The results were dismal.

> *Healthcare organizations have done a poor job of engaging their physicians. Few physicians are emotionally bonded and loyal to the organizations they work for, according to Gallup's 2005 physician database, which contains aggregated ratings of healthcare facilities across the country. At the 50th percentile of the database (facilities with average overall ratings),* **only 10% of physicians are fully engaged***, while 38% are actively disengaged. That's nearly a 4-to-1 ratio of antagonists to advocates.*

> [*Can Hospitals Heal Anemic Physician Engagement?* Rick Blizzard, The Gallup Organization, September 2005]
> http://www.gallup.com/poll/18811/can-hospitals-heal-anemic-physician-engagement.aspx

Furthermore, the survey found "physician ratings stems to some degree from the idea that in highly rated facilities physicians feel like they 'fit,' both from an emotional standpoint (physicians feel proud to be associated with them) and from an operational standpoint (physicians feel the organization is perfect for physicians like them)."

So, what is to be done? How can we improve the state of physician engagement in our healthcare institutions?

The folks at Gallup had some preliminary recommendations, beginning with operational basics:

- The ability to manage emergencies
- The efficiency of the admission process

- The quality and timeliness of radiology
- Surgical scheduling

When healthcare organizations meet these basic expectations, they help establish a good fit for their physicians.

But operational efficiency is not enough. In our work, we find organizations must also foster strong relationships between physicians and other staff members, starting at the top. They must establish a shared purpose with common goals like improved patient satisfaction and clinical outcomes.

Most importantly, to build physician engagement, trust has to be nurtured between physicians, administrators and staff at every level.

In 2013 another study by Canadians on physician engagement revealed that "physician engagement does not happen on its own."

[*Exploring The Dynamics Of Physician Engagement And Leadership For Health System Improvement: Prospects for Canadian Healthcare Systems,* ed. Lori Anderson, Canadian Foundation for Healthcare Improvement, April 2013]
http://www.cfhi-fcass.ca/sf-docs/default-source/reports/Exploring-Dynamics-Physician-Engagement-Denis-E.pdf?sfvrsn=0

According to this study, organizations must use diverse strategies and initiatives to strengthen physician engagement and leadership, including (but not limited to):

- **Physician compacts** as mechanisms that help clarify roles, expectations and accountabilities between physicians and other system leaders

- Leadership that is linked to broader improvement strategies to create a receptive context for physician engagement in improving clinical outcomes

- **Leadership development**—especially for collective and distributive leadership—to support physician engagement

- **Teams and team leadership**—especially inclusive leadership—as a favorable context for physician engagement and leadership, and performance improvement

The concept of "burnout" is a relatively new one in the annals of human history. Peasants, in medieval times, for example had no such concept. You worked or you were in serious trouble. It is only after two World Wars and the 1960s that human beings start finally experiencing burnout.

Clinical psychologist **Herbert Freudenberger** first identified the construct "burnout" in the 1970s.

Along with his colleagues, Freudenberger theorized the burnout process can be divided into 12 phases (not necessarily followed sequential). Many victims of burnout skip certain stages; others find themselves in several at the same time and the length of each phase varies. [*Burned Out*, Ulrich Kraft, *Scientific American Mind*, June/July 2006 p. 28-33]

1. **The Compulsion to Prove Oneself**: Often found at the beginning is excessive ambition. This desire to prove oneself while at the workplace turns into determination and compulsion.

2. **Working Harder**: Because they have to prove themselves to others or try to fit in an organization that does not suit them, people establish high personal expectations. In order to meet these expectations, they tend to focus only on work while they take on more

work than they usually would. They may even become obsessed with doing everything themselves. This will show they are irreplaceable since they are able to do so much work without enlisting the help of others.

3. **Neglecting Their Needs**: Since they have devoted everything to work, they now have no time and energy for anything else. Friends and family, eating and sleeping start to become seen as unnecessary or unimportant as they reduce the time and energy spent on work.

4. **Displacement of Conflicts**: Now, the person has become aware that what they are doing is not right, but they are unable to see the source of the problem. This could lead to a crisis and become threatening to oneself. This is when the first physical symptoms are expressed.

5. **Revision of Values**: In this stage, people isolate themselves from others. They avoid conflicts and fall into a state of denial towards their basic physical needs while their perceptions change. They also change their value systems. The work consumes all energy they have left, leaving no energy and time for friends and hobbies. Their new value system is their job and they start to be emotionally blunt.

6. **Denial of Emerging Problems**: The person begins to become intolerant. They do not like being social and if they were to have social contact, it would be merely unbearable for them. Outsiders tend to see more aggression and sarcasm. It is not uncommon for them to blame their increasing problems on time pressure and all the work they have to do, instead of on the ways they have changed.

7. **Withdrawal**: Their social contact is now at a minimum, soon turning into isolation—a wall. Alcohol or drugs may be sought out for a release since they are obsessively working "by the book." They often have feelings of being without hope or direction.

8. **Obvious Behavioral Changes**: Coworkers, family, friends and other people that are in their immediate social circles cannot overlook the behavioral changes of this person.

9. **Depersonalization**: Losing contact with oneself; it's possible they no longer see themselves or others as valuable. The person also loses track of their personal needs. Their view of life narrows to only seeing in the present time while their life turns to a series of mechanical functions.

10. **Inner Emptiness**: They feel empty inside and to overcome this, they might look for activity such as overeating, sex, alcohol or drugs. These activities are often exaggerated.

11. **Depression**: Burnout may include depression. In that case, the person is exhausted, hopeless, indifferent and believes there is nothing for them in the future. To them, there is no meaning of life. Typical depression symptoms arise.

12. **Burnout Syndrome**: They collapse physically and emotionally, and should seek immediate medical attention. In extreme cases, usually only when depression is involved, suicidal ideation may occur with it being viewed as an escape from their situation. Only a few people will actually commit suicide.

A study funded by the American Medical Association and the Mayo Clinic found 45.8% of respondents reported experiencing at least one symptom of serious burnout, such as emotional exhaustion, depersonalization and a low sense of personal accomplishment. [*Burnout and Satisfaction With Work-Life Balance Among US Physicians Relative to the General US Population*, Arch Intern Med/ Vol 172 (No. 18), October 8, 2012]

Of the surveyed physicians, the study compared 6,179 practicing doctors ages 29 to 65 with 3,442 workers of the same age group in other fields. Doctors had a higher risk of emotional exhaustion (32.1% versus 23.5%) and overall burnout (37.9% versus 27.8%).

The report **defines burnout** as a syndrome characterized by a **loss of enthusiasm for work** (emotional exhaustion), **feelings of cynicism** (depersonalization) and a **low sense of personal accomplishment**. Burnout may erode professionalism, influence quality of care, increase the risk for medical errors and promote early retirement. Burnout also seems to have adverse personal consequences for physicians, including contributions to broken relationships, problematic alcohol use and suicidal thoughts. Incidentally, the term "burnout" was identified 30 years ago to describe "a state of fatigue and frustration among health and service workers arising from excessive demands on their resources." Sound familiar?

If anything, the rapid pace of change in the healthcare industry will lead to an even higher incidence of burnout. The rising demands for care from aging baby boomers and a projected 30 million newly insured patients under the Affordable Care Act will only make this dire situation worse.

Why Do Physicians Shy Away from Leadership?

According to a study by McKinsey (*When Clinicians Lead*, McKinsey Quarterly, February 2009), there are several factors that encourage physicians to shy away from leadership roles:

- Ingrained skepticism among clinicians about the value of spending time on leadership. We usually hear physicians saying, "I am already a leader."

- Financial disincentive (loss of income)

- Negative peer recognition for reducing clinical practice to take leadership role

- "Going to the Dark Side" perception by peers for taking leadership roles

- Lack of supporting and nurturing development culture

- Physician bias and culture

In addition, through our work with physicians, we find the following additional factors that encourage physicians to shy away from leadership roles:

- **Unfamiliarity:** Leadership and management is not their core competencies, and is not their comfort level

- **Lack of Talent Management and Succession Planning:** In 2009, we conducted a survey of succession planning in healthcare and discovered healthcare lags many other industries in succession planning. In fact, we found no published evidence of physician succession planning.

- **Avoidance Due to Stress:** Leadership roles come with stress and headaches due to the need to have uncomfortable conversion with peers and the need to deal with disruptive behaviors.

- **Generational Differences:** After seeing their parents spending lots of time away, the younger generation of physicians value their personal time with family and value less the need to spend time in serving on committees and being in meetings.

- **Lack of Capacity and Time:** Today, healthcare organizations can no longer afford to send physicians to generalized leadership development workshops, hoping for substantial outcomes. In an era of WRVU, physicians cannot afford the lost productivity by traveling to leadership conferences.

- **Lack of Applied Learning**: "I went and got an MBA and none of the case studies were healthcare!" one physician told me.

- **Cultural Factors:** Lack of alignment between "expert culture" and "collective culture."

What people don't realize is the vast differences between collective and expert cultures leads to tension, conflict and stress; especially if we lack alignment and purpose.

Most healthcare professionals are acclimated to a collective culture, whereas physicians belong to an expert culture. In the former category are such professionals as nurses, therapists, administrators and support staff. These professionals usually work in groups, tend to avoid conflict and are not high risk-takers. Physicians, in contrast, tend to be individualistic risk-takers who prize their autonomy.

Outside of patient care, they are more likely to be motivated by self-interest than by group values.

- **Traditional Leadership Training Falling Short:** Some leadership training programs still teach the traditional model of leadership—a hierarchical pyramid, with the CEO at the top taking decisions and then passing them down a chain for implementation and execution. The top-down approach has long proven anathema to a physician "expert" culture immersed in providing answers to patients.

- **Current Medical Education Curricula Ignores Leadership Skills:** A majority of physicians, as many as 70% according to a University of South Florida survey, very early in practice felt their education ill equipped them to realize their full worth citing ignorance in leadership development, difficulty working with others, ineffective communication, disengagement with their patients, amongst other attributes.

A study showed there was a significant drop off in patient empathy between the 1st year of medical school and the 3rd year. In its conclusion, the study noted this decline was reversible and suggested medical schools introduce targeted educational programs to cultivate empathy and improve clinical outcomes. *[An empirical study in decline of empathy in medical school,* M.Hojat et al., Med Educ, 2004 Sep 38(9): 934-941]

Physicians were inadequate when it came to influencing others, delegating tasks, communicating with non-medical staff, ensuring quality control, generating strategy, displaying financial and business acumen, driving effective change, building trust, creating succession and focusing on patient centered care.

The diagram below shows the holistic view taken by the Physician Leadership Institute when it comes to physician development.

We used a checklist of desirable attributes under the domains of professionalism, business, clinical and people skills and found that between medical training and the credentialing process, *none were covered.*

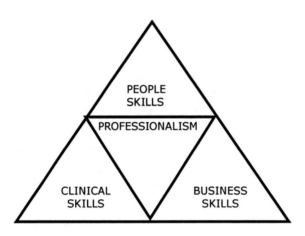

Dr. Lennox Hoyte at University of South Florida College of Medicine tells us the problem is built into the very nature of medical school training:

> Traditional medical training *is based on the idea of becoming the best individual, becoming masters in our specialties. This training process was designed for a time when physicians ran the healthcare enterprise, and everyone accepted healthcare to be an extremely hierarchical arrangement, with doctors sitting on the top of the pyramid. And this is something we have been taught all our lives. The traditional system was based on the master-apprentice approach, where seniority*

conferred authority.

Let me explain: As a student, you start by getting the best grades so you can be the top of your class to create the most competitive medical school application. You work hard to differentiate yourself, and demonstrate your uniqueness. In medical school, you work hard again to be at top of your class, so you can be picked by the best residencies. Then, predictably, you're trying to be the best resident, in order to be accepted at your chosen fellowship, or land the best job. Then you go for a fellowship, and guess what – you're trying to prove that you're the best fellow. This sequence does not naturally lend itself to the kind of training required for leadership.

For me, leadership entails something entirely different. It's about inspiring individuals to work together to achieve amazing results. It is about bringing ordinary people together to accomplish extraordinary things. The leader is not the one with the best ideas, but rather the person that inspires others to come up with the best ideas, and choose the ones that are suitable for solving the problem at hand; to obtain agreement among team members and stakeholders, and to guide the team so that they obtain the desired results. In so many ways, I see leadership as the job of inspiring others to achieve, to fire them up, and aim them at the problem to be solved. It requires an unselfish mindset that puts the team and project first. That's quite a different mindset from what we are taught in the traditional path of medical training.

Physician leadership can be taught, and this teaching must encompass the entire career, starting with medical school, and continuing through clinical training, and lifelong professional education after formal training is completed.

Like clinical specialists, we, at the Physician Leadership Institute, believe future generations of physicians will be **Lea-derists**™ i.e., the physicians who combine clinical skills with leadership skills to achieve transformational results that benefit the patient.

Why Physician Leadership Matters

The lack of trained physician leaders might explain why healthcare continues to be at the crossroads, unable to chart a vision for this millennium, plagued with inconsistent and uneven quality of care, mired in cost overruns, underachieving results that don't match investment and a physician workforce which feels disconnected from patients and the organization.

However, when physicians turn their energy and attention to providing leadership, the results are nothing short of transformative.

The Benefits of Collaborative Leadership
A hierarchical, sequential model of leadership that promotes top-down decision-making through the CEO or a Chief Medical Officer is not the best way to introduce physicians to leadership roles.

Instead, leadership should be distributed as envisioned by a study commissioned by McKinsey in collaboration with the London School of Economics, which assumes a more distributed look (See our modified diagram).

[*When clinicians lead*, James Mountford and Caroline Webb, *McKinsey Quarterly*, February 2009]

http://www.mckinsey.com/insights/health_systems_and_services/when_clinicians_lead

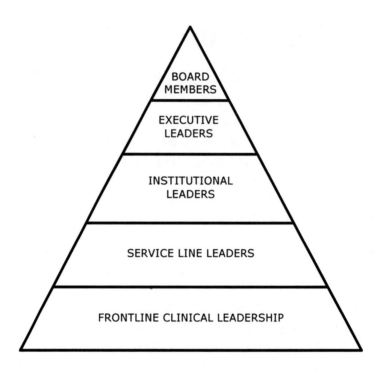

As the diagram shows, they propose a tiered structure that provides for distinct categories of leadership.

At the top, **institutional leaders** who give the organization its broad strategic vision and use their clinical skills along with their administrative and leadership expertise to realize and communicate the vision. Due to these qualities, these leaders provide the critical interface between the rest of the organization and those with executive and financial control.

In the middle, **service line leaders** who are heads of their units or departments, passionate about the healthcare provided by their specialties but also imbued by the values and needs of the organization. They are driven by innovation and are result oriented. In the trenches, **frontline clinical leaders**, not only possessing great clinical skills for direct delivery of healthcare to the patients but also seek constant improvement in care as one of the organization's values. In this structure, leader is not a stagnant honorific given to some, kept from many; instead **leadership is a thoughtful and systematic process, a journey, even part of the culture's DNA**.

These three levels are distinct yet closely interlocked and whilst institutional and service line leaders might assume a greater overall responsibility, it is the more numerous frontline clinical leaders tasked with their day-to-day experiences to inform and guide the improvement of services and realize the organization's vision.

Why is this so important? The same study found UK hospitals that engaged their physicians in active leadership roles **improved their performance by 50%** in key areas as compared to peers with low physician participation.

Similarly, in the U.S., high performing medical centers achieved their results immersing their physicians in leadership collaborations with administrators, emphasizing clinical quality and innovation. [Stephen M. Shortell et al., *"An empirical assessment of high-performing medical groups: Results from a national study,"* Medical Care Research and Review, 2005, Volume 62, Number 4, pp. 407–34; Lawrence Casalino et al., *"External incentives, information technology, and organized processes to improve health care quality for patients with chronic diseases,"* Journal of the American Medical Association, 2003, Volume 289, Number 4, pp. 434–41]

A distributed leadership model proves attractive to physicians because it exposes them to a level of leadership that relates to their strength. A frontline physician with strong clinical skills but not necessarily invested in giving the organization its strategic vision will find more resonance in taking the lead in ensuring quality care on a daily basis. The more ambitious physician who has a feel for where the organization should be heading might find the mantle of strategic leader more appealing and fast track as an institutional leader.

In the 90s, Kaiser Permanente Colorado was struggling with poor clinical and financial performance while losing doctors to rivals. Desperate to turn things around, they recruited Dr. Jack Cochran, a pediatric plastic surgeon as executive medical director. Within five years, Kaiser's Colorado affiliate had become the healthcare organization's shining star in quality of care and profitability, an example to be followed by others.

Cochran's mantra of clinician as *"healer, leader, and partner"* suffused the organization, bringing everyone on the same page: *To provide leadership in ensuring improvement in patient outcomes. Patients left significantly more satisfied, physician retention improved dramatically, and financially Kaiser Colorado zoomed from zero to $87 million in income.* [*Innovation In The Kaiser Permanente Colorado Region,* Bill Marsh MD and David Price MD, Perm. J, 2005 Fall, 9(4): 40-43]

The Veteran's administration system of hospitals faced similar problems in the mid-90s with poor performance threatening its closure. At stake, the health needs of hundreds of thousands of retired military veterans.

Enter Dr. Kenneth Kizer, an emergency medicine specialist, emphasizing clinical leadership throughout the organization. Under his leadership and vision, the VA reorganized into 21 centers of excellence, stressing patient care and measurable outcomes. Improvement was financially incentivized, pay for performance was introduced and medical informatics introduced to improve documentation and record progress.

The results: The VA brought mortality rates down 40% in men aged 65 and over category as compared to the national average. Satisfaction rose to 83%, a 12% increase over U.S. levels, as the number of VA patients doubled over the following decade. [Ken Kizer: Transforming The VA, *Medsphere,* 2013]

In each of these examples and others, doctors took the leadership role in improving clinical services, not as a one off project but by changing the culture of the organization.

Through collective accountability and professionalism of clinicians coming together to achieve one goal, ensuring the delivery of excellent and timely patient care, clinicians collaborated with administrators on important clinical decisions such as resource allocation and reconfiguration of clinical services in a symbiotic manner. In addition to clinical outcomes, the deeper overall quality of the patient experience was what mattered to these physician leaders.

Each department or clinical service performance was tracked in real time and lapses were not brushed aside but studied for further improvement. In a sense, there was osmosis of a clinician's sense of responsibility for his patient to the organization itself.

This is a central theme in physician leadership: ***alignment with the organization's values and vision.***

Rx: THE PRESCRIPTION

Defining Physician Leadership

When I ask a room full of physicians what is Physician Leadership, I get a wide range of answers. Leadership means different things to different people, thus the first step of physician leadership transformation is to be grounded in the distinction of physician leadership.

In his book *Nicomachean Ethics*, Aristotle establishes that an ethical leader is *"one who nurtures members of an organization to realize their own potential."*

While we can't all receive instruction from Aristotle, his principles live on to this very day. In today's U.S. Army, a **leader** is:

> *...anyone who by virtue of assumed role or assigned responsibility inspires and influences people to accomplish organizational goals.*

And in today's medical field, one only has to talk to physicians like Dr. Lennox Hoyte to learn the same lesson.

> *I remember how we participated in a specific workshop with the Physician Leadership Institute in which we were challenged to find a solution to a problem. The team stood around in a circle and tried to accomplish the challenge, with modest success. No one was speaking up. It occurred to me that, as individuals who are trained to be right, physicians face an element of risk in voicing ideas or opinions that may be wrong. This leads many to avoid speaking up unless they are 100 percent certain that they are right. But this is not the way that unbelievably amazing things get accomplished.*

Amazing things get accomplished when we start out with less than perfect ideas and progressively improve them to get to the results we want to achieve.

I realized then, that the job of the leader is to "make it safe to speak up." I offered a few suggestions, which were not very good ones, but what I learned and witnessed, was that the initial, modest ideas led others on the team to offer progressively higher quality ideas.

Soon, we were hearing ideas from everyone, and the best solution came, unexpectedly, from the physician who was the quietest one in the room.

It's like when you gather around and ask your friends to start telling jokes. The first jokes aren't very funny, but then people loosen up and start telling funnier and funnier jokes. The leader is the one who breaks the ice and makes everyone comfortable.

The job of the leader is to inspire others to achieve. From Alexander the Great to today's leaders that has not changed.

At this point, let's look at the definition of leadership itself. It is instructive to note the U.S. Army view:

Leadership is the process of influencing people by providing purpose, direction, and motivation while operating to accomplish the mission and improving the organization.

Again, this may seem like common sense, but it is a far more complex topic because leadership is not about definitions; instead it is about a state of being and about actions with others to accomplish a specific mission or goal.

The Army's **BE-KNOW-DO** model of leadership is a proven leadership framework:

> *Army leadership begins with what the leader must BE—the values and attributes that shape character. It may be helpful to think of these as internal and defining qualities possessed all the time. As defining qualities, they make up the identity of the leader.*
>
> *The knowledge that leaders should use in leadership is what Soldiers and Army civilians KNOW. Leadership requires knowing about tactics, technical systems, organizations, management of resources, and the tendencies and needs of people. Knowledge shapes a leader's identity and is reinforced by a leader's actions.*
>
> *Leaders cannot be effective until they apply what they know. What leaders DO, or leader actions, is directly related to the influence they have on others and what is done. As with knowledge, leaders will learn more about leadership as they serve in different positions.*

[BE-KNOW-DO, Leadership The Army Way, Leader to Leader Institute, Jossey-Bass, 2004]

In the field of healthcare, however, there are specific weaknesses that must be addressed. As mentioned earlier, physicians are trained to "DO." They are not trained to be BE nor KNOW others to engage them collaboratively. Being empathetic and building relationships has not been historically emphasized.

Thus, our definition of physician leadership must look something like this:

> **Physician leadership is a role (not a title) that provides purpose and vision to *inspire, engage and influence people to collaboratively deliver tangible results.***

Guided by the above definition, the shift in paradigm from physician and physician leader becomes clearer:

From Physicians	To Physician Leaders
Autonomous care providers	Collaborative, team-based care
Practice advocates	Organization or team advocates
1:1 Interactions, instant gratification	1:N interactions, delayed gratification
Reactive philosophy	Proactive philosophy
Deciders/doers	Delegators/planners and designers
Knowledge holders	Coordinators of knowledge (Quarter back)
Resistant to change	Embrace and lead change
Conflict and risk-avert	Skilled negotiators, produce 'win-wins'
Follow directives	Set vision and energize others
Play not to lose	Play to win

Table 1: The shift from physician to physician leader

The Physician Leadership Model™

The **Physician Leadership Model** was developed, tested, validated and refined by the Physician Leadership Institute (PLI) and includes key competencies and observable behaviors physician leaders are encouraged and expected to demonstrate on a consistent basis in a specific clinical team, organization, culture or community.

We organized the leadership competencies and behaviors around the **five disciplines of Leading with Purpose, Leading with Strategy, Leading Self, Leading People** and **Leading for Results.**

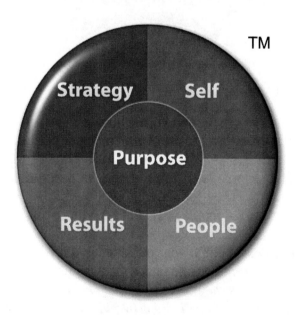

The Physician Leadership Model

Leading with Purpose

"Efforts and courage are not enough without purpose and direction."
- *John F. Kennedy*

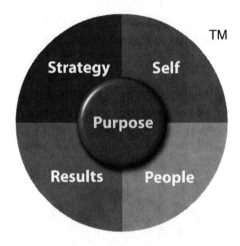

Powerful leaders create and communicate meaning—connecting employees at every level to the overall purpose of their work.

Leaders align people with the mission, values and the vision of the organization. They tell us why we do what we do, what the organization and its people stand for, and where they are going.

In *The Art of War* (a 3,000 year old strategy book), Sun Tzu placed the "Tao" as the number one factor for a leader's success. Sun Tzu said: *the Tao causes the people to be fully in accord with the leader, thus they will die with him; they will live with him and not fear danger.*

Dave and Wendy Ulrich, co-authors of *The Why of Work* remind us: *In organizations, meaning and abundance are more about what we do with what we have than about what we have to begin with* (2010, p. 27). At the Physician Leadership Institute, we help organizations and their leaders articulate their purpose by answering the following questions:

- **Mission:** Why do we exist? What is our purpose as an organization? The department? The individual? Do we live by our mission in our day-to-day activities? Do we understand the patient is our reason for existence?

- **Values:** What do we hold in high esteem? What do we stand for? What will we not do? Is how we do our work as important as what we do?

- **Vision:** Where are we are going? How do we get there?

- **Performance:** How will we know we are succeeding? How do we measure improvements? How do we reward performance?

- **Alignment:** Does everyone in the organization believe in the mission? Do we uphold and act on the values of our organization? Are we aligned to the vision? Do we share a common sense of purpose, responsibilities and outcomes? Are we working collaboratively across departments and functions to achieve our common goals?

Profit, as Peter Drucker points out, cannot be a reason for existence. Instead, he says:

> *The customer is the foundation of a business and keeps it in existence. He alone gives employment. To supply the wants and needs of a consumer, society entrusts wealth-producing resources to the business enterprise.* [*Management: Tasks, Responsibilities, Practices;* Peter Drucker, p.61]

The physician leader must have a clear purpose and narrative for his/herself. *Why do I get up in the morning? Why did I get into medicine?* It is the lack of clarity of purpose that leads to frustration, stress and burnout.

In addition, the physician leader speaks with purpose to inspire team members to come together and solve problems in a collaborative way. A shared purpose gives team members a sense of belonging and motivates them to act in order to achieve positive outcomes.

Leading with Strategy

"The effective strategist (leader) only seeks engagement after the victory has been won, whereas he who is destined to loose first fights and afterward looks for victory." *-Sun Tzu, The Art of War*

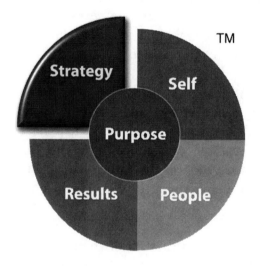

Beginning with the organization's purpose, strategy is about selecting the best choices about the future—for the organization, employees and the transformational physician leader.

James Mountford and Caroline Webbin, *When Physicians Lead* (McKinsey Quarterly, February 2009) define a physician leader as one able to "communicate a powerful, clinically based vision and have deep, broad skills in both leadership and administration.

"These skills are both 'hard,' such as strategic thinking and planning, and 'soft,' such as negotiation and influence."

Healthcare and Financial Perspective

The physician leader thinks and acts like an owner. They understand the changing landscape of business issues and their implications on their practice and organization, and are financially literate. The sweeping changes triggered by the Affordable Care Act (ACA) make this a required leadership attribute.

Strategic Thinking and Terrain Mapping

The physician leader continuously assesses the healthcare terrain, explores strategic choices and communicates the vision, goals and priorities to the team members. They know choosing what *not do* is as important as what we choose *to do*.

Systems Thinking

The physician leader understands systems consist of people, structures and processes that work together to make an organization "healthy" or "unhealthy." The physician leader presents a unified vision of the future and follows a consistent pattern of purpose, embodying the vision in their everyday actions.

Leading Change

The physician leader is a catalyst of change. They are agile and comfortable with ambiguity during the healthcare paradigm shift. The physician leader effectively assesses stakeholders' level of support or resistance and is able to influence them without formal authority.

Innovation

The physician leader is an innovative and integrative thinker, challenging the status quo, often taking two different and opposite options together and forging the best out of each for a unique solution. They align the need for change with the capabilities of the team and individuals, and lead by example.

Evidence-Based Decision Making

The physician leader makes evidence-based decisions and does not delay decisions. They are strong proponents and practitioners of Evidence-Based Medicine.

Leading Self

"Knowing others is intelligence; knowing yourself is true wisdom. Mastering others is strength; mastering yourself is true power."
-*Tao Te Ching*

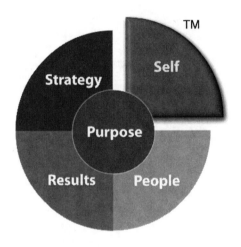

Before you can lead others, it is essential to know and lead oneself.

As Tao states, in order to unleash the full potential in others, you first have to unleash your own potential to the fullest. Transformational physician leaders are authentic by seeing and knowing themselves first, then seeing and leading others.

Peter Drucker states: *We must be our own CEO.* [*Managing Oneself,* Peter Drucker, *Best of HBR,* 1999] To do that successfully we have to know our strengths and weaknesses, our learning style, how well we work with others, what are our values and in what areas can one contribute the most. One of the most important ways one can ascertain strengths and weaknesses is to employ feedback assessment, like a 360-degree assessment.

When important decisions are made, record your expectations and then 9 months to a year later, match it up with actual results. Drucker practiced this for years and he called it one of the cornerstones to being a successful leader. Feedback reveals your strengths, skills that need strengthening, skills needing delegation, disruptive bad habits and requisite socialization needed to achieve results.

Knowing who you are allows you to paradoxically reveal your vulnerabilities to your colleagues, which in turn builds trust.

A CEO who shows he's not a morning person or is somewhat disorganized will find more people willing to make accommodations. Robert Goffee and Gareth Jones, in their provocative *Why Should Anyone Be Led By You*, discovered successful CEOs found "sharing an imperfection effective because it underscores a human being's authenticity." [*Why Should Anyone Be Led By You*, Robert Goffee and Gareth Jones, *Harvard Business Review*, Sept –Oct, 2000]

Another advantage is it pre-empts inventing one by colleagues who as per human nature are suspicious of anyone who projects themselves as flawless. The keyword is selective – weaknesses should not jeopardize your professional role or prove fatal to the organization.

Goffee and Jones also emphasize: *Leadership must always be viewed as a relationship between the leader and the led... there are no universal leadership characteristics. What works for one leader will not work for another.*

Thus a leader will continuously assess the needs of their followers and modify their leadership approach appropriately to:

- Deploy their personal values, strengths and even weaknesses to maximize their effectiveness as leaders

- Understand and integrate inherent tensions of leadership

- Size up situations and adapt their leadership behavior without losing their unique differentiators to drive results

Organizations must help leaders realize the importance of managing their energy levels. This is a critical skill for all healthcare practitioners, regardless of position.

Engaging others to make positive changes in their organizations starts with leaders who:

Lead Self
- Are self-aware
- Pursue purpose with a passion
- Model the way by clarifying personal values and aligning their actions with their values
- Lead with their hearts as well as their heads
-

Then Lead People
- Seek to understand the needs and concerns of others
- Embrace and inspire a shared vision with exciting possibilities for all involved
- Establish enduring relationships
- Build trust, garner support, establish collaborative goals and share power

As part of our **Physician Leadership Model,** the attributes of leading self, include:

Integrity and Excellence
The physician leader exhibits integrity in all actions, deeds and

intentions. They model organizational values in their day-to-day behavior, setting the example of excellence for all around him or her.

Adaptability and Agility
The physician leader adapts easily and quickly to change; is versatile and open to new ideas. Innovation and agility in decision-making are hallmarks of true leadership. Their goal is to find solutions, not assign blame.

Emotional Intelligence
As part of our Physician Leadership coaching, we work with physicians to hone the so-called "soft skills."
Daniel Goleman calls these attribute emotional intelligence:

- *Self-awareness*—knowing one's strengths, weaknesses, drives, values and impact on others

- *Self-regulation*—controlling or redirecting disruptive impulses and moods

- *Motivation*—relishing achievement for its own sake

- *Empathy*—understanding other people's emotional makeup

- *Social Skill*—building rapport with others to move them in desired directions

The physician leader is aware of strengths and weaknesses, shows candor and demonstrates composure in adversity. They can control their disruptive emotions and impulses. They are highly motivated, show empathy and possess superior social skills. For many physicians, these are serious weaknesses that in the past have prevented them from becoming organizational leaders.

Life-Long Learning

Today's environment of constant change shows the necessity of keeping an open mind. The physician leader constantly challenges and develops. They learn from others and from their own mistakes, and seek feedback at all levels of the organization—directly and indirectly.

Courage

The physician leader has the intellectual courage to confront difficult problems and challenges, making tough decisions while considering the organizational and human impact of their decisions. Performance and courage are often inextricably linked.

Energy and Optimism

The physician leader maintains a high energy level that energizes others. In our Physician Leadership Institute, we introduce physicians to four dimensions of personal energy—physical, emotional, mental and spiritual. Because their followers often emulate a leader's mood and attitude, it is critical to always demonstrate a contagious enthusiasm, optimism and a can-do attitude across all activities and situations.

Leading People

"A leader is best when people barely know he exists, when his work is done, his aim fulfilled, they will say: we did it ourselves."
- *Lao Tzu*

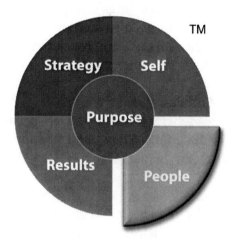

Daniel Goleman says the best leadership blend comes when the authoritative "Come with me" combines with the affiliative "People come first." The first states the end but empowers people with the means to that end while the second builds relationships and with that harmony, loyalty and flexibility.

Trust-based Relationships
The physician leader is dependable, treats others with respect and builds trust through everyday actions. The physician leader relates well to people at every level by showing consideration and empathy. Their attitude and demeanor motivates fellow workers and colleagues.

Effective Communication

The physician leader keeps everyone well informed. They express ideas clearly and spend considerable time listening. They ensure the mission of the organization is clearly understood by their teams. They are often gifted storytellers who can inspire others with a sense of purpose and direction.

Coaching and Performance Improvement

The physician leader helps others improve their performance by providing timely and constructive feedback. They show appreciation for a job well done and coach the team with empathy and by setting high performance standards.

Teamwork and Collaboration

The physician leader is a team player collaborating across departments and functions. They build high-performance teams by bringing out the best in members.

Empowering Others

The physician leader matches the right job to the right person, empowering others to take responsibility and manage their work with self-confidence.

Conflict Management and Negotiation

The physician leader seeks win-win solutions and is always open to criticism. They are inclusive in asking for opinions and feedback, and are capable of viewing issues from multiple perspectives.

Leading for Results

"The Pinnacle of excellence is not marked by number of the victories, fame for wisdom or courageous achievement, it is about flawless execution." - *Sun Tzu*

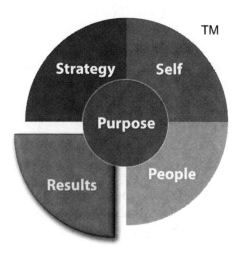

The essence of results is a prediction, a look into the future. With it comes uncertainty. Successful leaders are prescient, looking to the future and assessing the present to measure the alignment or gap between a desired result and what they have at the moment. They then reduce the variables by shrewd resource allocation, measuring performances, ensuring best practices, emphasizing customer satisfaction, seeking innovation and motivating everyone to be on the ball with the big picture.

Achieving the right results in a timely fashion is the *raison d'etre* of being a leader.

There has never been a bigger wakeup call than the Health Age for prospective physician leaders. They stand at the cusp of a revolution and these are the things they need to do.

Patient Focus
The physician leader is focused on patient (customer) needs. They respond to patient concerns with empathy and kindness. Timely communications and a sense of "caring" are critical tools in helping physicians bring their patients a sense of comfort and confidence.

Quality and Process Improvement
The physician leader focuses on improving work processes to provide higher levels of quality, reduce waiting times, as well reducing costs and eliminating waste. The "customer experience" is an important work-process that is always part of the leader's agenda.

Driving Results
The physician leader leads by being accountable and holding others accountable for the timely and quality delivery of care. They avoid procrastination and exhibit a purposeful sense of urgency.

Safety and Technology
The physician leader maintains safety standards, using technology effectively to empower their teams and enhance productivity.

Productivity and Efficiency
The physician leaders know time is precious. They plan and lead productive meetings, manage time effectively and minimize the disruption of busy schedules.

Doing Right Things and Doing Things Right
This is a cliché, perhaps, but applicable on a day-to-day basis for the physician leader. Results-driven leaders, by default, create a high performance culture. Another point to note: physician leaders do focus on measuring outcomes but not at the expense of quality or consideration for the patients.

Why Leadership Development Programs Fail

The January 2014 issue of the *McKinsey Quarterly includes a timely discussion on four common, avoidable* mistakes that companies make in the implementation of their leadership programs [*Why leadership-development programs fail*: Pierre Gurdjian, Thomas Halbeisen, and Kevin Lane, *McKinsey Quarterly* , January 2014]:

  1) Overlooking context
  2) Decoupling reflection from real work
  3) Underestimating mind-sets
  4) Failing to measure results

The Physician Leadership Institute addresses each one of these pitfalls in the very design and execution of our physician leadership sessions. Let's examine each of these in detail.

Context
According to the McKinsey article, too many training initiatives rest on the assumption one size fits all and the same group of skills or style of leadership is appropriate regardless of strategy, organizational culture or CEO mandate.

Here's how the author frames the context debate:

> *In the earliest stages of planning a leadership initiative, companies should ask themselves a simple question: "What, precisely, is this program for?" If the answer is to support an acquisition-led growth strategy, for example, the company will probably need leaders brimming with ideas and capable of devising winning strategies for new or newly expanded*

business units. If the answer is to grow by capturing organic opportunities, the company will probably want people at the top who are good at nurturing internal talent.

Focusing on context inevitably means equipping leaders with a small number of competencies (two to three) that will make a significant difference to performance. Instead, what we often find is a long list of leadership standards, a complex web of dozens of competencies and corporate-values statements. Each is usually summarized in a seemingly easy-to-remember way (such as the three R's), and each on its own terms makes sense. In practice, however, what managers and employees often see is an "alphabet soup" of recommendations. We have found when a company cuts through the noise to identify a small number of leadership capabilities essential for success in its business—such as high-quality decision making or stronger coaching skills—it achieves far better outcomes.

In our experience, the best approach takes context into account in its very design. Our Physician Leadership institutes and academies are built around the observed challenges in the field. And to make sure the focus is on the right challenges, participants have to undergo a 360-degree assessment before they start our programs. The assessment is used to tailor sessions for each participant, ensuring the team curriculum is balanced with individualized dimensions.

Decoupling from Work
The author's view is presented as follows:

When it comes to planning the program's curriculum, companies face a delicate balancing act. On the one hand, there is value in off-site programs (many in university-like settings) that offer participants time to step back and escape the pressing demands of a day job. On the other hand, even after very basic training sessions, adults typically retain just 10 percent of what they hear in classroom lectures, versus nearly two-thirds when they learn by doing. Furthermore, burgeoning leaders, no matter how talented, often struggle to transfer even their most powerful off-site experiences into changed behavior on the frontline.

The answer sounds straightforward: tie leadership development to real on-the-job projects that have a business impact and improve learning. But it's not easy to create opportunities that simultaneously address high-priority needs—say, accelerating a new-product launch, turning around a sales region, negotiating an external partnership or developing a new digital-marketing strategy—and provide personal-development opportunities for the participants.

Our Physician Leadership Institute approach does both. We start by first building up the foundational attributes of physician leadership, using our **Physician Leadership Model**. This is followed by action projects where cross-functional teams embark on their challenge projects—fixing some of the organization's most pressing concerns. The impact of these "action learning" projects, allows the physician leader to "be-know-do" in ways tied directly to business performance.

Mind-sets

Change won't happen if minds don't change. Here's how the issue is described in the McKinsey article:

Becoming a more effective leader often requires changing behavior. But although most companies recognize that this also means adjusting underlying mind-sets, too often these organizations are reluctant to address the root causes of why leaders act the way they do. Doing so can be uncomfortable for participants, program trainers, mentors, and bosses—but if there isn't a significant degree of discomfort, the chances are that the behavior won't change.

In healthcare, the issue is no different. A common response is as follows: *I am already a leader, why do I need leadership training?*

Our physician leadership programs are designed to change minds. The "expert" individual-contributor culture of the medical profession fosters individual leadership but fails at building organizational leaders. We help these "experts" step beyond their comfort zones to become organizational leaders.

Measuring Results

The final obstacle to change is lack of accountability. Here's how the article states the issue:

> *We frequently find that companies pay lip service to the importance of developing leadership skills but have no evidence to quantify the value of their investment. When businesses fail to track and measure changes in leadership performance over time, they increase the odds that improvement initiatives won't be taken seriously.*
>
> *Too often, any evaluation of leadership development begins and ends with participant feedback; the danger here is that trainers learn to game the system and deliver a syllabus that is more pleasing than challenging to participants. Yet targets can be set and their achievement monitored. Just as in any business-performance program, once that assessment is complete, leaders can learn from successes and failures over time and make the necessary adjustments.*

The article goes on to suggest an important way to measure the efficacy of leadership training:

> *One approach is to assess the extent of behavioral change, perhaps through a 360 degree–feedback exercise at the beginning of a program and followed by another one after 6 to 12 months.*

At the Physician Leadership Institute, we use this 360-feedback approach, coupled with another performance-based metric—the *actual ROI* of the action-learning projects commissioned through our programs. This allows all involved to see the impact of physician leadership at both individual and organizational levels.

Finally, we make sure our physician leaders understand the transformation is a journey that never ends. All our programs include an ongoing leadership component that ties back to the organization's strategy and purpose.

Lasting success requires leadership development that is well-targeted, high quality, delivered on-site and customized to the needs of physicians and the organization. The goal is to transform physician leadership at all levels and build the next generation of physicians who can successfully lead healthcare transformation.

I'd like to propose one more reason for why leadership development programs fail—*culture.* Too often, change programs are implemented without adequate organizational support.

Ask yourself:

> - How do we design, foster and nurture the right culture for our organization?
>
> - How do we build the right organizational "habits" that exemplify this culture?
>
> - How do we define what behaviors are not culturally acceptable? What must change?
>
> - How should our leaders model the behaviors?
>
> - How do we align everyone—at all levels—in the organization?
>
> - Is our culture scalable and sustainable?

- How does investing in our leaders contribute to transforming our culture?

By providing compelling reasons for the organization's existence, a leader builds a narrative capturing the imagination of all stakeholders—from the patients who are receivers of care, to the providers themselves—the clinical and nursing practitioners who serve the patient and society.

The Physician Leadership Journey: Identifying & Closing the Gap

So how exactly does transformation happen?

Transformative learning is defined as "a deep, structural shift in basic premises of thought, feelings, and actions." [Mezirow, J. (2000) *Learning as Transformation: Critical Perspectives on a Theory in Progress.* San Francisco: Jossey Bass]

At the core of transformative learning is the process of "perspective transformation" with three dimensions: **psychological** (changes in understanding of the self), **convictional** (revision of belief systems) and **behavioral** (change in lifestyle).

An important part of transformative learning is for individuals to change their frames of reference by critically reflecting on their assumptions and beliefs and consciously making and implementing plans that bring about new ways of defining their worlds.

This process is fundamentally rational and analytical. Learning can be divided into four stages. [In the Mush, Flower, J., *Phys Exec*: 1999 Jan-Feb;25(1):64-6]

1. **Unconscious Incompetence**: The individual does not understand or know how to do something and does not necessarily recognize the deficit. They may deny the usefulness of the skill. The individual must recognize their own incompetence and the value of the new skill, before moving on to the next stage. The length of time an individual spends in this stage depends on the strength of the stimulus to learn.

2. **Conscious Incompetence**: Though the individual does not understand or know how to do something, he or she does recognize the deficit as well as the value of a new skill in addressing the deficit. The making of mistakes can be integral to the learning process at this stage.

3. **Conscious Competence**: The individual understands or knows how to do something. However, demonstrating the skill or knowledge requires concentration. It may be broken down into steps and there is heavy conscious involvement in executing the new skill.

4. **Unconscious Competence**: The individual has had so much practice with a skill it has become "second nature" and can be performed easily. As a result, the skill can be performed while executing another task. The individual may be able to teach it to others, depending upon how and when it was learned.

Fitts and Posner [Magill RA. *Motor Learning and Control*: Concepts and Applications. 2007] also posited early learning was characterized by a high degree of **cognitive activity** requiring extra-ordinary levels of attention with performers being inconsistent and typically committing a number of errors without knowledge of how to correct them.

This early learning is extremely mentor-heavy, requiring plenty of demonstration and feedback. The early phase was replaced by an **associative intermediate phase** with performers becoming more consistent and requiring less attention, more proficient in error detection and correction as they develop an internal model.

The last stage, **the autonomous stage** is when the performer was most proficient and efficient, made strategic decisions, multi-tasked and could easily correct the few errors that occurred. Very little attention or cognition is required at this stage and the skill is executed as "second nature" (i.e., mostly through unconscious or sub-cortical processes).

The **Physician Leadership Model** developed by the Physician Leadership Institute (PLI) incorporates the features of transformative learning and the four stages of competency, or skill acquisition. The model also avoids the caveats of the cottage industry of instant and ineffective remedial leadership fixes by focusing on transforming the personal DNA and meshing it with the organization for physicians to become part of the leadership culture.

We offer a comprehensive fellowship program onsite which extends to a year in line with the Accreditation Council for Graduate Medical Education (ACGME).

Participants are trained in capabilities that go beyond their clinical skills such as:

- Collaboration (versus Competition)

- Adaptability to Rapid Change

- Win-Win Negotiations

- Team Based Clinical Care

- "We" versus "I"

- Organizational Alignment

- Business and Financial Skills

- Creativity

- Risk Taking

The goal of the Physician Leadership Institute (PLI) is to transform the leadership capabilities within an organization at all levels.

We aim to equip leaders with cutting edge leadership tools and practices, enable participants to engage in team collaboration and provide them access to an elite team of facilitators. The curriculum is comprehensive, multi-faceted and comprised of fully customized sessions based on the specific leadership needs of the organization and the incoming cohort.

PLI encompasses a range of teaching modalities, including in-depth case analysis, individual and small group learning, teamwork, interactive lectures and discussions, application based reading and related assignments, action learning projects, group simulation activities, personal reflection activities, mentoring and coaching.

We believe every organization has unique culture and leadership needs, that is why we customize the curriculum and the structure (at 5 levels) aimed at practically transforming the DNA of physician leadership:

1. The program is customized to meet the organization's strategies and needs. (What skills do you need your leaders to have to help you navigate current and future healthcare challenges and achieve your vision?)

2. The curriculum is customized again to the cohort baseline assessment results based on their top development areas identified in the 360° assessment.

3. The learning and coaching is customized thereafter to the individual leader based on their individual needs and development plan.

4. The physician led projects are customized and aligned to the organization's strategic plan and priorities.

5. The individual sessions are customized with the organization's real life case studies to make it relevant.

Similar to clinical fellowships accredited by the Accreditation Council for Graduate Medical Education (ACGME), the graduates of the PLI become fellows of the Institute. They are **Leaderists** who have undergone our transformative, total immersion fellowship program. The result is a balanced leadership style that combines technical knowledge with leadership skills along the five dimensions of our industry-leading **Physician Leadership Model**. It's about effectiveness (doing right things) and efficiency (doing things right) - with the heart and mind of a leader. Organizational alignment and performance are natural by-products.

At the Physician Leadership Institute, we have quantified the benefits of physician leadership measured by each of our clients. Our Physician Leadership Transformation journey is a process of continuous improvement.

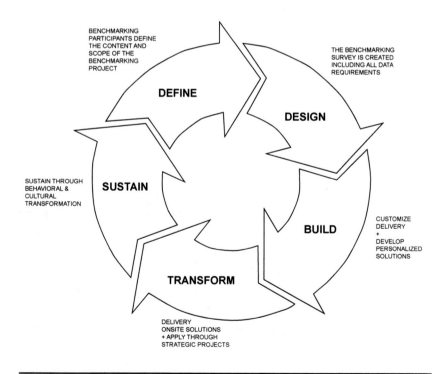

Assess

Working with our leadership assessment tools, we help you assess your challenges – both organizational and personal – establish measurable goals, evaluate existing gaps and identify priorities and opportunities.

Measure

We establish a baseline for key leadership performance indicators for your organization and build an evidence-based leadership performance system.

Build

Using the results from our evidence-based leadership assessment we work with you to customize a development structure and programs for your organization. The curriculum will use our tested delivery approach that includes customized topics, coach matching and team based applied team action learning projects designed around the specific challenges facing your organization and your team.

Transform

Our onsite solutions enable your entire organization to embark on the Physician Leadership Transformation Journey. Leadership metrics are based on outcomes. Your organization tracks progress and results over time.

Sustain

As the impact of our physician leadership program starts being felt in the workplace, we help you create an "evidence-based" monitoring system with key leadership metrics based on outcomes. These are the measurements you need to track progress and results over time. We also help you identify the next steps—the areas of strategic impact your organization needs to tackle next. As part of the cycle of continuous improvement, this is a critical component of physician leadership.

The 360° Assessment

The Leadership Transformation Journey is rooted in PLI's evidence based, best-practice, rigorous 360° assessment in which the physician assesses his or her strengths and weaknesses in the four leadership dimensions and then is assessed in turn by peers, the clinical staff, the management and others like students and patients to establish a baseline from which PLI can then customize the transformation experience through a series of training modules.

The Multi-Source Feedback (MSF) tool developed by PLI goes beyond the traditional clinical competencies assessments in vogue at hospitals and medical centers as it tests emotional intelligence, leadership traits, strategic vision and result-oriented behaviors. The 360° feedback is then compared to the physician's self-report and used to determine which dimension needs development in order to help improve the physician's identified weaknesses.

Recent meta-analysis of medical literature examining the impact of peer assessment and physician specific feedback showed an overwhelming 70% of studies demonstrate peer feedback's positive effect on clinical performance. [Veloski, JJ., et al., 2006, Systematic Review of the Literature on Assessment, Feedback, and Physician' Clinical Performance: BEME Guide No 7. *Medical Teacher* 28(2): 117-28]

More importantly, an extensive review of the conditions contributing to the effectiveness of 360° feedback showed organizational context, including the intentional and deliberate use of such MSF for developmental purposes rather than for promotion or financial recognition, contributed to its success.

Planned interventions after feedback, such as coaching, were important in effecting behavioral changes. [Atwater L., et al., 2007, Multisource Feedback: Lessons Learned and Implications for Practice. *Human Resource Management* 46(2): 285- 307]

There is also growing evidence that 360° feedback is most salient in highlighting weakness in "soft" skills or emotional intelligence which physicians seem to have the hardest time self-identifying [Tham, K., 2007, 360 Feedback for Emergency Physicians in Singapore. *Emergency Medicine* 24: 574-75] and MSF is more useful improving such skills than when used in relation to clinical competencies. [Sergeant, JK et al., 2007 Challenges in Multi Source Feedback: Intended and Unintended Outcomes, *Medical Education* 41: 583-91]

With the 360° tool, PLI can then customize a precise, results-driven transformation program, which includes the following components:

Data Driven Results
Every participant in PLI starts with a baseline of measured physician strengths and development areas based on a confidential, online 360° assessment of leadership skills and competencies.

These skills and competencies are re-measured six months after graduation to demonstrate sustainable learned behavioral change. PLI has documented a range of *60% to 200% improvement.*

Customized Curriculum
The Physician Leadership Institute curriculum is customized for each cohort's strengths and development needs as identified through the 360°assessment process.

Comprehensive Assessment
In addition to 360° assessment tools, PLI also relies on other gauges of leadership competencies: communication styles, transformation and change, business and financial acumen, stress, time management, trust, accountability, teamwork, performance management and conflict resolution. The information gathered from these assessments is used to create individual and team development plans.

Personal Development Plans

These development plans are aligned with individual purpose through the use of a PLI developed proprietary tool, the **Personal Strategy Map™** (PSM) to ensure each prospective physician leader is in control of his or her transformative journey. These maps identify the strengths and areas of development which are meshed with the physician's personal values and mission, and used to chart out realistic and measurable goals of behavioral change and personal development in an expected time frame.

Coaching

Participants are matched with a network of accomplished healthcare and business coaches to create and implement personal development plans. This partnership deepens the learning and behavioral transformation process and reinforces ownership of personal development.

Strategic Applied Learning Projects

Physicians have the opportunity to apply the leadership learning by working in cross functional teams to improve upon strategic, organization-wide issues and then drive tangible results for a return on investment. In addition, physicians learn the skills of strategic planning, collaboration, holding others accountable, having crucial conversations and execution towards a common goal. Each project team is assigned a project champion from within the organization senior leaders (sponsor) and a professional project mentor (coach).

Interacting, Networking and Working with Peer Physicians and Leaders

Given the active, participatory nature of the institute environment, learning with and from your classmates is one of the most important aspects of the program. Participants learn as much from each other as they learn from the faculty, thereby creating a strong support system and a network of colleagues and friends that will be sustained well beyond the institute experience.

Simulation-Based, Experiential Learning

PLI utilizes active, adult learning models along with simulation-based and experiential learning techniques. Participants are placed in real-life scenarios and are directly responsible for the changes that occur as a result of their decisions. Examples of such activities include an equine-assisted learning experience, an executive challenge (ropes) course, and financial and business simulations.

PLI has access to a stellar group of more than 75 national faculty members and industry leaders who contribute to the fellowship program, who are affiliated with University of South Florida, Duke University, Emory University, Harvard University, Stanford University, the U.S. Military Academy at West Point, Washington University in St. Louis, General Electric, Lehigh Valley Hospital and Florida Hospital, to name a few.

Emotional Courage

Researchers tell us why so many leadership programs fail: *Programs fail to teach emotional courage, the courage needed to stand up and speak your mind and to take ownership for decisions and actions. These acts provoke discomfort, anxiety, and uncertainty. The PLI engages emotional courage needed to lead through relevant and tangible projects which require risk taking and ownership of those decisions.*
We use retired military leaders from West Point to address and deal with emotional courage.

Alignment & Outcomes

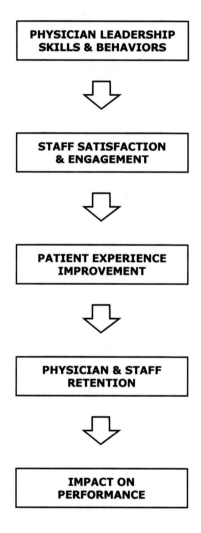

Our work at the Physician Leadership Institute is organized around outcomes that drive physician engagement and performance. Engagement does not happen overnight, to say the least. It requires an organizational commitment as well as individual commitment from all participants.

Today, healthcare organizations can no longer afford to send physicians to generalized leadership development workshops and hope for substantial outcomes. Lasting success requires leadership development that is well-targeted, high quality, delivered and embedded on-site and customized to the unique needs of physicians *and* the organization.

The goal is to transform physician leadership at all levels and build the next generation of physicians to successfully lead healthcare transformation.

How do we produce that alignment?

What people don't realize is the vast differences between collective and expert cultures lead to tension, conflict and stress, especially if we lack alignment and purpose.

Most healthcare professionals are acclimated to a collective culture, whereas physicians belong to an expert culture. In the former category are such professionals as nurses, therapists, administrators and support staff. These professionals usually work in groups, tend to avoid conflict and are not high risk-takers. Physicians, in contrast, tend to be individualistic risk-takers who prize their autonomy. Outside of patient care, they are more likely to be motivated by self-interest than by group values. In a recent USF survey, 70% of physicians felt they lacked leadership and organizational alignment skills. Many of them were averse to such alignment and felt it infringed on their autonomy and expertise.

The underlying factor in navigating through change in healthcare is to understand and bridge the differences between the expert culture and the collective culture through alignment.

Ask:

- How may we foster a culture that is less hierarchical and more patient-centric?
- How may we build a cross-functional understanding across departments?
- How may we understand what it means to be accountable to each other, as well as the patient?

Let's look at how we design a Model for Alignment. The key design principles are as follows:

The Alignment Model Must be Built on Shared Values and Purpose

Without a common purpose, no alignment model will succeed. What is critical is the process for creating the shared values must to some extent be collaborative and integrative. It is the heart of the transformation and cannot be rushed.

There are three levels of alignment that must be dealt with simultaneously:

Individual Alignment

This is an individual level alignment focused on helping the individual with their leadership strategy and development areas, usually identified using a 360° assessment. The physician works on their own individual development plan and on a biweekly frequency works on tangible actions to change their leadership behaviors.

Project Alignment

At any given time, the number of change initiatives in a health system is overwhelming. Project alignment is focused on helping participants solve assigned problems and guiding them through project, team dynamic and stakeholders buy-in. This should happen once or twice a month as a group. Project alignment drives accountability to deliver on the project commitments as well as teaches problem solving, project management and collaboration as a team.

Team Alignment
This is group coaching focused on helping the teams with their leadership gaps identified in the 360° and other assessments. Learning is key and teams build on their individual alignment objectives to create a shared experience as teams. Topics cover a wide range of leadership and team issues such as communication, collaboration, conflict, etc.

The Alignment Model Must be Based Upon the Hospital's Service/Practice Portfolio
The Alignment Model is based upon the actual services being delivered. To measure patient experience, performance, quality and costs, the model must be organized around the products or services provided to the customers, and then, one can calculate the cost per unit to deliver the service and the unit price to charge the customer for the service. This area is going to be a critical part of your competitiveness for the future.

The Alignment Model Should be Started and Focused Around an Immediate Major Initiative or Issue
The best way to start is to build alignment via action learning projects that have a major impact on the work flow of physicians and patients.

The Alignment Model Must be Data-Driven
The model cannot be static. It must dynamically capture performance data at a point in time and compare trends, changes and improvements toward targets.

The Alignment Model Must Maintain Financial Integrity

If the changes introduced by an Alignment Model can't be reconciled with real financial data, it will not be useful or taken seriously. There will be a glaring disconnect between talk and action.

The Alignment Model Must be Led by Physician Leaders

Physician leaders who have been certified as change agents are trained to understand the tools and tactics required to drive organizational change. They are certified in much the same way as a Six-Sigma team for change management. If the Alignment Model is not building physician engagement and enthusiasm, then it is not authentic and is wasting precious resources. Unfortunately, most institutions tend to see physician leadership as a title.

Where should your organization begin engaging their clinicians in the leadership of the organization and the initiatives? Who should they invest in to help lead?

Our answer is **leadership is not a title, rather, leadership must be everywhere in the organization**. Each one of us needs to lead from where we are. Leadership is not a program, a book or a retreat. Leadership is a thoughtful and systematic process, a journey, even part of the culture's DNA.

Typically, organizations tend to invest in clinicians already in leadership roles by sending them to various leadership conferences. But these clinicians typically account for less than 20% of the clinicians making a difference in the healthcare transformation.

The focus should be to invest and recruit the 80% of the clinicians who are in the trenches.

Case Study: The Iowa Clinic

Like many multispecialty groups, The Iowa Clinic is the product of practice mergers and consolidations. Despite transition over time from a "group of practitioners," the clinic's "one group" culture has remained its steadfast goal. To continue to thrive, The Iowa Clinic recognized the need to engage physicians as leaders throughout the organization's infrastructure. Enhancing its leadership strengths became a priority that would transform the clinic and prepare it for the future.

The Iowa Clinic consists of over 180 providers, made up of 150 physicians and 30 advanced practitioners. The clinic includes 8 primary practice locations in the Greater Des Moines area and over 30 outreach locations throughout Central Iowa. These locations accounted for over 500,000 patient visits this past year. It is the largest physician-owned multispecialty group in Central Iowa operating as a patient focused, physician-governed clinic. The Iowa Clinic aims to be the premier physician group of Central Iowa.

Mark Reece, M.D., The Iowa Clinics Chairman of the Board of Directors once said:

> *National healthcare reform will have far-reaching effects on efficient and effective healthcare delivery. The transformation that is occurring... requires us to take our leadership capacity to a higher level by focusing on, and providing additional skills and leadership tools that are beyond clinical skills.*

Traditionally, physicians are groomed to be domain experts in their respective fields, devoting their focus and energy to providing high-quality clinical care. They are "doers" who dedicate themselves to the one-on-one patient interaction, obtaining near-instant gratification in their jobs. Being successful necessitates autonomy and elicits independence to treat patients effectively. As a result of their education and traditional practice background, these "practice advocates" identify themselves as medical professionals first and foremost and often perceive responsibilities that don't directly relate to clinical practice as extraneous and unnecessary. This was especially true for many physicians at The Iowa Clinic.

Recognizing the changing healthcare environment, with declining reimbursements, increased competition and consolidation, The Iowa Clinic sought to improve physician engagement. Trust and communication were indispensable elements in the successful relationship between administrators and clinical operators. As such, The Iowa Clinic predicted that improving the leadership skills of their physicians would translate to reduce variations, improved quality, enhanced strategic planning and improved outcomes. As a result, the Board of Directors decided to invest in its physicians and administrators by building a leading physician leadership development program. After evaluating various options, the board elected to partner with the Physician Leadership Institute (PLI) in Tampa, Florida, which offers leadership development programs customized to the unique needs of the organization and its leaders. The 12-month onsite curriculum included personalized coaching, group-based strategic projects and onsite experiential and simulation-based sessions. The goal of PLI's program was to transform the "DNA" of The Iowa Clinic's leadership at all levels by creating a strong, unified vision fully capable of fulfilling the clinic's mission and goals. A key strategy was to engage physicians in driving the transformation of The Iowa Clinic into the leading physician group in Central Iowa.

Since its establishment in 2010, The Iowa Clinic's Physician Leadership Institute has graduated more than 70 leaders. For the inaugural class, 17 physicians and leaders were selected through a comprehensive nomination and review process. The first class consisted of 11 physicians spanning 10 specialties, 2 board members and 4 administrators, including the clinic's Medical Director. The second cohort of 16 physicians and administrators included 3 board members. The third and fourth cohorts consisted of more than 40 physicians who had recently joined The Iowa Clinic.

Program participants underwent a comprehensive 360° assessment, receiving honest and confidential feedback from their peers and direct reports from key stakeholders on 55 leadership competencies and behaviors. The 360° assessment was administered prior to the program launch to identify individual and group strengths and needs, and was also delivered at the program's completion to measure improvements. Top initial strengths of the group included leading through personal excellence and integrity, decision-making and sound judgment, analytical and critical thinking, and maintaining quality and customer focus. Development areas included managing conflicts by accepting constructive feedback and negotiating with others, leading change and innovation, and developing and communicating a clear vision to create engagement. This was an eye-opening experience as many physicians received this type of feedback for the first time.

Monthly program sessions such as: The Art of Terrain-Based Strategy, Leading with Courage, Leading Self then Leading Others, Creating and Maintaining High-Performance Teams, and Process Efficiency were mostly scheduled for afternoons and evenings to preserve productivity. A variety of teaching modalities, including simulations, group discussions and case analyses, maintained participant engagement throughout the program. Faculty included military leaders, healthcare futurists, dean of academic medicine and authors. In addition, the institute held bi-monthly one-on-one coaching meetings where a trained, professional coach was matched with each participant based on their needs that were identified in the 360° assessment.

One of the Physician Leadership Institute's many success stories is from a practicing surgeon. Similar to other physicians, he entered the program believing he was already a leader who understood his clinic's needs and not needing any form of formal leadership development. Before the program, he was quoted saying, "Empathy is for people with free time," and "I'm not here to be your friend."

As he continued in the program, this physician learned about his leadership style and how he related to others. As a result of the lessons learned from the sessions, project and coaching, his perceptions and values changed. During the program, he created a personal strategy map and was part of the project tasked with creating a physician-led organization. His interactions with peers taught him that not everyone operates in the same manner and being an effective leader requires self-knowledge and collaboration. Currently, he considers "listening" his most important leadership skill and values his relationship with his team. Since his graduation, he was promoted to Chief of Surgery, an accomplishment he self-attributes to the continued application of leadership skills acquired during the program.

Physician engagement requires practice. The clinic's board created opportunities for physician engagement by selecting projects that strategically impacted the clinic's culture, strategic direction, and service line. Physicians and administrators got engaged by working in cross-functional teams as part of the leadership program to address the challenges presented to them.

In one engagement opportunity, the team was asked to research what the "Physician Led Organization of the Future" would look like given all the changes in healthcare. The team built a business strategy and plan that included a market analysis, best practice benchmarks and multiple recommendations for strategic implementation. During their project, members were tasked with comprehensively considering, evaluating and aligning all of The Iowa Clinic's options, including hospitals, accountable care organizations (ACOs), and multiple standalone multispecialty groups.

Another Iowa Clinic top priority was to transform its Cardiovascular Service Line by improving quality outcomes, increasing patient volume and reducing costs. To accomplish this, the team assessed and identified workflow efficiency and optimization as well as communication and marketing strategies. The successful implication of their project increased cath lab handling volume from 45% to 64%, adding 200 patients and $114,000 in annual revenue. Inpatient cardiology and cardiovascular cases rose from 56% to 72%, an increase of 240 admissions and $170,000 in revenue.

Another project identified by The Iowa Clinic was to improve patient experience and create a patient focused culture. Team participants were tasked with creating a process that assessed, measured, reported and rewarded patient satisfaction. Key deliverables included a new survey tool, data management processes and an administrative process (including follow-up) that clearly established service standards. As a result, a Customer Service Standards Handbook was created based on The Iowa Clinic's five core values: "Friendliness, Respect, Teamwork, Ownership, and Excellence." The Handbook was associated with a patient-focused culture road map, training plans and event kickoff to energize staff and providers.

As a result of these projects in the leadership program, physician engagement spread beyond the structured leadership institute. Physicians and leaders became passionate about the key strategies they developed such as patient experiences. For example, Christina Taylor, M.D., a Physician Leadership Institute graduate engaged in the patient experience project, became the Chief Quality Officer for the Iowa Clinic, championing patient experience and patient outcomes.

Graduates' engagement in the Physician Leadership Institute continues as they become mentors for new recruited physicians. Physician hands-on mentoring is already leading to better cultural integration and accelerating success for the new physicians.

Leadership development programs are linked to increased physician satisfaction and engagement, improved direct reporting job satisfaction and organizational alignment, and improved quality and safety metrics.

Graduating classes from The Iowa Clinic's Physician Leadership Institute produced tangible improvements in each participant. Sample reported results (high % ability before and after):
- 133% improvement in the ability to lead others.
- 200% improvement in the ability to work in teams.
- 350% improvement in the ability to think strategically.
- 167% improvement in the ability to effectively communicate and influence.
- 325% improvement in the ability to deal with difficult issues and situations.
- 150% improvement in the commitment to and active engagement in ensuring TIC's success.
- 250% improvement in loyalty to the organization.

Statistical analysis of both pre and post 360° assessment data demonstrates statistical evidence ($p<0.05$) that physician leadership competencies and behaviors have improved as assessed by others. The most improved competencies were strategic thinking, managing conflict, team development and collaboration, and leading change and innovation.

Most telling was the answer to this question:

Would you recommend participation in the Physician Leadership Institute to other physicians?

100% of the respondents said, "Yes."

The Iowa Clinic Physician Leadership Institute continues to be a transformational journey, enriching its participants both professionally and personally. The development program has tangibly benefited the physicians, The Iowa Clinic, its patients and the surrounding community. Several graduates have received promotions and recognitions in testaments to its success. Similarly, since completion of the first class in 2011, the clinic has run three additional cohorts in its ongoing commitment to excellence. Additionally, many other Iowa-based organizations have adopted physician leadership development programs similar to The Iowa Clinic's Physician Leadership Institute. One example is the Physician Leadership of Iowa sponsored by the Iowa Hospital Association in partnership with the Physician Leadership Institute.

C. Edward Brown, The Iowa Clinic CEO attributes the clinic's ability to change with agility and speed to engage physician leadership: *Our investment in physician leadership has helped us to develop the skills and talents among physicians to adjust organizationally during these dynamic times.*

Daniel Kollmorgen, M.D., a practicing Iowa Clinic surgeon, perhaps put it best: *My key takeaways from the Institute experience were that leadership is about listening, relationships, and self-awareness. These skills are not necessarily developed or maintained in our practice of medicine. I believe the future of medicine will depend on us as physician leaders who can look beyond their daily routines, understand and apply leadership concepts in patient care, administrative roles, and in our personal lives.*

Case Study: The Physician Leadership Institute of Ohio

The Ohio State Medical Association (OSMA) and the Ohio Hospital Association (OHA) engaged the Physician Leadership Institute (PLI) to create the Physician Leadership Institute of Ohio (PLIO) with the mission to develop physician leaders in Ohio.

As Ohio's first and only statewide physician leadership development program, the PLIO had a goal of developing cultures of team leadership in hospitals and health systems that include skilled physician leaders. This innovative program provided the Ohio physicians with a forum to become transformational leaders in clinically integrated delivery systems across the state.

This unique collaborative effort has improved leadership skills in the area of physician hospital relations, team management, care coordination and population health management. Its creation is the product of physician leaders and hospital administrators committing to empowering physicians with the knowledge, skills and experience to provide more than clinical care and to become dynamic leaders in integrated delivery systems.

The program teaches physicians to lead with strategy by working with their teams and hospital partners to identify and implement strategic and clinically integrated population health initiatives. It helps physicians learn to lead people through this period of uncertainty and change in our healthcare delivery system. And it helps physicians lead for results by maximizing performance of their clinical teams, optimizing safety and enabling their groups and organizations to thrive in the new healthcare environment.
The Physician Leadership Institute of Ohio has engaged more than

50 physicians with 12- 20 physicians per institute. Each of these institutes has provided an individualized and comprehensive assessment of each physician's skills at the beginning and end of the program to ensure improvement in leadership skills, knowledge and experience.

The PLI experiential approach immersed the physicians in 4 key areas: seeing self-first as leaders, inspiring their teams, leading change strategies and delivering transformative outcomes. This innovative approach develops hospital and health system physician leaders in a collaborative manner with the medical society and hospital association. It is a commitment by the state physician leadership and hospital administrators to promote physician hospital relations in a transformative and positive way.

A graduate of the Ohio program notes:

> *The Physician Leadership Institute has taught me that doctors can work together in a collegial manner to help shape healthcare reform, rather than just waiting to react to the change and hope to survive.*

This is a testimonial, not only to the effectiveness of our approach, but is in fact a testimony to the organizational commitment to cultural transformation.

The PLI Ohio graduates reported the following **high impact improvements**:

- 200% improvement in the ability to **work collaboratively in teams**
- 80% improvement in the ability to **think strategically**
- 100% improvement in the ability to **communicate and influence**
- 200% improvement in the ability to **deal with difficult issues/conversations**

- 67% improvement in the ability **to accept their role as a leader**
- 100% improvement in the **ability to work with the executive team**
- 133% improvement in the **willingness to be engaged in the organization**
- 400% improvement in the **willingness to serve in a leadership capacity**
- 60% improvement in the **ability to impact patient satisfaction**
- 50% improvement in the **ability to increase quality and improve clinical outcomes**
- 80% improvement in the level of **their work satisfaction**

Most telling was the answer to this question:

Would you recommend participation in the Physician Leadership Institute to other physicians in Ohio?

100% of the respondents said, "Yes."

Interviews: Perspectives on Physician Leadership

While perspectives on the status of physician leadership vary from practice to practice, the underlying message is surprisingly consistent. We've included the voices of several healthcare practitioners here in the form of interviews.

The questions we asked them were all related to the topic of physician leadership.

We're grateful to the following leaders for their thoughtful insights:

- C. Edward Brown
- Dr. Daniel Kollmorgen
- Ed Lopez
- Dr. Lennox Hoyte
- Dr. Joe Cooper

INTERVIEW WITH C. EDWARD BROWN

The Iowa Clinic is a $120-million, fully integrated multispecialty clinic with more than 140 physicians and healthcare providers practicing in 32 specialties. The group has about 500,000 patient visits each year, 167,000 of whom are unique patients.

The Iowa Clinic also enjoys national influence thanks to its involvement with the American Medical Group Association (AMGA). Its chief executive officer, C. Edward Brown, has served as a past chair of AMGA and has been a member of the board for 10 years.

You've been at The Iowa Clinic for a considerable time. As the leader of the organization, what are the biggest challenges you face?

The biggest challenge is that of adapting to the demands of the industry to remain relevant as we create the new delivery systems for healthcare services. Our culture has to rapidly adapt to change to improve our service.

We know that the old model of governance is no longer sufficient – we need more physician engagement in the decision-making process. If our change initiatives are to succeed, we found out that we need physicians to *not just participate, but lead*. That's the only way to see results.

How do you find these leaders? How do you develop them?

We made a commitment to a five-year process for leadership development. Looking around, we wanted to build a stronger culture where we develop our leaders internally. We found Mo Kasti and The Physician Leadership Institute by circumstance – when we learned what they had done at the University of South Florida. Two things stood out: 1) the embedded nature of onsite learning, and 2) the experiential learning process, where leaders developed their talents by working on self-assessments to determine their leadership styles, then working on meaningful corporate projects that have a return on investment to the organization. Upon completion, these projects are delivered as formal reports to The Board of Directors and then implemented. The Iowa Clinic was the first in Iowa to establish an internal physician leadership institute. The entire program has had a dramatic change on the participants, and at a board level, we see a positive cultural change in the organization.

How does your organization create alignment between strategy and execution?

The Physician Leadership process has dramatically strengthened our culture and improved our ability to adapt to change because we have *"physicians leading physicians."* We have dramatically improved our internal capabilities. There are so many change imperatives and initiatives that our folks have had to embrace and they have done so because as we know, "culture eats strategy for breakfast." When physicians develop answers together, they build solutions even as they strengthen their own relationships amongst each other. They believe in the mission because they own it. The ability to execute becomes exponentially greater when you have a strong bond of trust in a common culture, a common way to doing things together.

There is no gamesmanship. Our physicians are extremely comfortable expressing their concerns openly. We focus not on blame, but on the outcome. For me this has been a personal journey over the last twenty years. We are a family of friends with a supportive culture that is, in many ways, the antithesis of the Fortune 500 model of competition. Our default mode is collaboration. That's the most powerful type of alignment.

What business impact do you get from this investment in physician leadership?

Physician leadership allowed us to make strategic moves that required extraordinary courage. We have been bold enough to do things that otherwise might appear unattainable. We have made these changes very rapidly, without the typical emotional stress that such changes cause. We have added many physicians to the organization and the Physician Leadership Institute is a mentor to them, helping them grow in our culture, nurturing the next generation of leadership. That is one of our cultural differentiators. Our physicians make the organization better for the future.

The result is that we have been successful in implementing lean process improvement through a holistic way of looking at healthcare – *population healthcare management.*

Our job is to serve the entire population in such a way that we prevent symptoms *before* they occur. We do the right thing focused on the patient. So to keep the patient healthy, we have a health coach for them, we make sure they have their medications on time and we make sure to see them in a timely manner – scheduling their visits. Our healthcare coaches follow up with their panel of patients to keep them abreast of their appointments, medications, and exercises. It's a "life panel."

What advice do you have for other healthcare executives as they face the organizational challenges of the future?

A few points: 1) *Embrace change* with courage. 2) Develop leaders who take individual responsibility in a team atmosphere. 3) Administrators must work for the physicians. I have 180 bosses – we work with each physician to make a difference and do our best for the patient. 4) Select your physicians carefully to make sure they will thrive in your collaborative culture, and finally, 5) instill a heightened sense of *stewardship* and of *ownership* of the process amongst the physicians.

INTERVIEW WITH DR. DANIEL KOLLMORGEN

Dr. Daniel Kollmorgen is a surgical oncologist, practicing with The Iowa Clinic in Des Moines. A graduate of the Physician Leadership Institute, Dr. Kollmorgen is the medical director of the John Stoddard Cancer Center.

How do you view physician leadership? Can physician leadership be taught?

I think the definition of leadership is evolving. The various forms leadership can take is one of the things I relearned in the year-long Physician Leadership Institute sessions with Mo Kasti. *What does it mean to be a leader?* It's not always the visible, captain-of-the-ship leading the charge.

There are a lot of different ways to lead and I think that is what is important today. Some people have different skills, but leadership is not just stepping up to be the CEO. It can be applied at every position and the best leaders adjust to each situation.

How does physician leadership impact work performance? Have you changed how you behave?

I think empathy from a leader is as important as command and control. When I'm in the OR, it's the captain-of-the-ship model, the buck stops with me. But I've learned the importance of relationships; being correct every time is not as important as maintaining relationships.

Relationships build success for the long run. How do you help others get to their goals? In the leadership class I learned about myself and how I'm perceived, and it's not the same for everyone. I became far more aware of how others perceive me, getting feedback on how my actions impact the team.

Self-awareness is huge, especially when you are in a leadership role where people might be intimidated by your position. You have to hold yourself back and remind yourself to be a friend, a teacher or a father. By encouraging others to participate and engage, you build a team for the long run. You have to learn how to switch hats – I have good days and bad days. Taking the leadership class improved my leadership skills and self-awareness, but it doesn't provide a foolproof formula.

Who should be enrolled in physician leadership?

I think there are significant benefits to wide participation. First, there's succession planning. Leaders need to be developed from within the local medical profession. Secondly, and more importantly, is the common language we share which comes from sharing the learning experience. We build a common lexicon and experience, which helps align us across different specialties and areas. You get a better understanding of where everyone is coming from, even if you don't use their strategy.

The spillover into your personal life is significant as well. Trust is a relationship-building tool across all human interactions. The journey is about going from being "unconsciously incompetent" to "consciously incompetent" and then slowly evolving and becoming "unconsciously competent." I'm still catching myself as I fall back into old habits.

How has physician leadership impacted your business?

The biggest difference has been the breaking down of silos across our multi-disciplinary group. At the board and committee level, we've shared common experiences that brought us all closer together as individuals.

We're not just business associates and partners, we're friends. We've built shared values and experiences. I have a better understanding of the colleagues in my class. I recognize how important group activities and culture building is in the greater scheme of things. We've built a stronger business culture, with a common vision, a common purpose; that's powerful. It's helped make the big business decisions less difficult – you don't have to go to the wall to get 100% input on every decision. We trust each other to do the right thing in ways we probably would not have earlier.

Is physician leadership a prerequisite for navigating the turbulence in the industry?

If physicians want to maintain or have any say in the future direction of healthcare, they are going to have to see the bigger picture. If you can't lead, engage and participate, you'll become just a cog in the wheel. I think that physicians know what's best for the patients and that without physician leadership we won't be able to make our voices heard. Physician leadership can eliminate barriers between disciplines and the administration. Again, the importance of relationships cannot be stressed enough.

INTERVIEW WITH ED LOPEZ

An '82 graduate of the University of Washington School of Medicine's Physician Assistant program, Ed Lopez later completed his formal internship and residency in general and specialty surgery at the Albert Einstein College of Medicine and Montefiore affiliated Hospitals in New York City.

After 17 years in private Cardiothoracic surgery practice and later as a co-founder of one of the largest private hospitalist programs in the country, Ed returned to business school completing his studies in professional medical management and healthcare policy at the University of Washington and the Harvard Kennedy School in Cambridge, Mass. Today as an Assistant Medical Director for a large healthcare system in the West, Ed is also a recent graduate of The Physician Leadership Institute's program in leadership sponsored by the Catholic Health Initiative (CHI). Ed has dedicated his efforts to mentoring, teaching and supporting young physicians to become the leaders of today and tomorrow in making the U.S. healthcare system the finest in the world.

In your practice, how do you define physician leadership?

I've done over 30 years in healthcare and over 20 of those years in staffing, managing physician practices, helping hospitals get the right contract surgeons, turning around failing practices and leading lean and process improvement projects in and out of hospitals. Those 30 years have shown me that *physicians are primarily technical experts* and frequently were never taught how to understand, empathize and motivate others. College and medical school were geared to a system of identifying high achieving individuals who, by themselves, could handle the most intense and arduous of demanding professions. And once the individual excellence was identified, they were often the most singly rewarded.

Most physicians were never formally taught to lead teams or

performance groups when they completed their training. Remember, we were training scientists, with the manual skills of DaVinci and the brilliance of Einstein. In fact, most, once finishing training, went into a practice and hired the talent that did that "organizational and management stuff" while they dedicated themselves to practicing the "art and the science of medicine."

But that was yesterday's model physician.

Today the need for physician leadership has never been more pronounced. As the 21st century healthcare culture and process of care delivery has changed, it has been wandering in the desert of darkness, looking for true leadership. And as we have seen when there is a void in leadership, there is never a shortage of politicians, policymakers, MBA's, economists and well-intended do-gooders filling that void. But for healthcare, it is not enough for physicians to be mere participants in the new system. Today the demand and the stakes are so high, that *only* the well trained and well-tuned physician leader can lead us through this healthcare change process successfully.

When did you first realize the need for physician leadership in the workplace?

I've been a big fan of Daniel Goleman and his concepts of emotional intelligence from the very beginning – for almost 20 years. But here's when it struck me in a way that could not be denied. I had gone back to grad school for a policy class – at the Kennedy School at Harvard – where at least one-third of my class was comprised of physicians, lawyers and policy makers from the rest of the world. I noticed that the behavior of the U.S. doctors was unique. We were technocrats, but not people or team leaders. The others were not just physicians in the office or the hospital. Rather, they were spiritual, community leaders as well. They were most often an integral part of the network of their community – not only as "medical healers," but they were also looked upon as social leaders who were involved in every aspect of their cultures. We, as healthcare delivery providers/physicians in the U.S., pride ourselves as specialists, sub-specialists and so have compartmentalized our profession that we have little to no say in our society anymore. We are looked upon as mere workers in the vast network of skilled professionals with no voice in the shaping of the future of our new healthcare culture. It was then that I realized that the physicians in this country were in trouble.

What happened? How did you go back to work and what were you thinking?

When I went back and started talking to my colleagues, they had never thought about it as I did. Most didn't care, as long as they were getting paid handsomely. The mindset was something like: "I'm responsible for hip surgeries. That's what I do and I do it well. I have a great referral base so I'm fine thank you very much. Don't bother me with this touchy-feely political stuff."

The result of the isolationist-specialist mindset is what you see in healthcare today. In the late 90s, we saw fresh-faced MBA's with no medical experience come into our healthcare systems and start dictating how business was to be run. Even then, the standard response was: "As long as they leave me alone to do my job and I get paid well, I won't get involved."

So healthcare issues have built up over time...

Sure, the history of our profession will show that until very recently, physicians had abdicated their responsibilities—perhaps not intentionally, but systemically. And in the mid-2000s, not only did physicians lose their say in healthcare, but they were at the mercy of a system that did not put the patient first. The few physicians who were in administrative positions were window dressing. They'd go to meetings and "participate" – not as physicians, but as cogs in the wheel. Physician leadership was non-existent. Unfortunately, they were neither physicians, nor leaders but mere participants in the vast healthcare machine. Some of us were thinking, "What have we created?"

That sounds bleak. Are things changing? Are physicians getting back into the game?

Thank God things are changing. Today, physicians are recognizing that there is a dearth of physician leadership at almost every level. The physician leader must understand today how the business works, what the outcomes are, how to lead and inspire teams, and fix problems – all from the perspective of the patient.

The government has stepped in as well – forcing the hospital systems to measure outcomes, not just costs. This is changing the business dynamic by forcing a sense of accountability for all of us – Doctor, Patient, payer, and administration. We *ALL* now own this thing called the American Healthcare system—you can run, but you can't hide.

To compete, our medical practices must nurture real, authentic physician leaders. Men and women, who understand that before we can lead others, we must search our souls and learn to lead ourselves in order to become the leaders we need to be. Leaders must inspire followers through servant leadership—by example and by service. No job is too small or too insignificant when it comes to the patient experience.

Can you give us an example?

There was a rural hospital with 25 beds that was a challenge because it was underperforming at nearly every metric used to measure performance.

The difference was physician leadership. We handpicked the physicians with the right emotional intelligence and with the leadership skills to succeed. Two of the physicians were new grads, another was a veteran, very discouraged and near the end of his career. We asked them if they wanted to make a difference. The veteran got behind us when he understood that this is why he had gone to medical school all those years ago. The right people make all the difference and this case was no different.

Today that hospital is the crown jewel in a 7-hospital system. We are getting results – focusing on outcomes and profitability. Morale is high and our patients love us.

You ask for a personal commitment from your physicians?

Absolutely, yes. My commitment is to do the right thing to help the patients and their families receive the finest experience they can have. No detail is too small. And we teach this to all – from the physician to the janitor. If a patient needs something, we do our best to get it for them. We tell them, "If anything isn't working for you, please let us know, so we can help."

There is science behind this. When a patient experiences a feeling of trust and faith, endorphins kick in and they begin their journey of healing with a positive frame of mind.

Look at what the patient experience is like in a typical hospital. The first thing we do is ask the patient to take off their clothes, wrap them in a piece of cloth and call it a gown with their butts hanging out. Strangers walk in and out of their rooms at all times of the day and night without a sense of privacy. They ultimately feel humiliated, confused and afraid, and yet, we expect them, when asked, to give that hospital a glowing rating when HCAHP scores come a calling. Is that any way to treat the patient?

Patients want and deserve to receive the best service in town while they are sick and hurting. The experience for the patient must be one they will feel comfortable with. We try to make it as much like a home as possible.

The patient experience is all-important?

It's everything. At our facility we have built a collaborative care model with the patient at the center. On daily rounds, physicians visit with all members of the staff who interact with the patients – nurses, therapists, discharge personnel, house-keeping – to ensure that we are all on the same page and understand the needs of the individual patient. No task is beneath anyone. We are butlers and servants. We are here to serve the patient, not pamper them, but rather to give them the respect they deserve. Humility is expected from all.

And the end result is patient satisfaction. Our patients ask to come back to us because they trust us.

This, by the way, is the best way to maximize shareholder value. By focusing on the best outcomes for our patients with results-driven leadership, that's physician leadership.

I have tried to live by and gain strength from an adage by Lao Tzu: *A leader is best when people barely know he exists, when his work is done, his aim fulfilled, they will say, we did it ourselves.*

INTERVIEW WITH DR. LENNOX HOYTE

Dr. Lennox Hoyte is a board certified OB/GYN physician and fellowship-trained in Urogynecology and Female Pelvic Medicine and Reconstructive Surgery. He treats women with prolapse, bladder and bowel incontinence, overactive bladder, childbirth related pelvic floor injury and complications related to vaginal mesh surgeries. He offers a wide range of successful surgical and nonsurgical therapies to treat these problems, specializing in advanced robotic surgery to correct vaginal prolapse, and is one of the leading robotic prolapse surgeons in the world.

In addition to his role as a clinician, Dr. Hoyte is active in the development of intellectual property related to the practice of medicine; he has filed and obtained U.S. patents on devices ranging from bladder drainage aids, to instruments for enabling prolapse surgery, as well as methods for accurately measuring intravascular blood volume. He is also Chief Medical Information Officer for the USF Physicians group, tasked with designing an electronic health record optimized for delivering high quality healthcare outcomes, while decreasing the documentation burden on providers.

How do you view physician leadership? Can physician leadership be taught?

Traditional medical training is based on the idea of becoming the best individual, becoming masters in our specialties. This training process was designed for a time when physicians ran the healthcare enterprise and everyone accepted healthcare to be an extremely hierarchical arrangement with doctors sitting on the top of the pyramid. And this is something we have been taught all our lives. The traditional system was based on the master-apprentice approach, where seniority conferred authority.

Let me explain. As a student, you start by getting the best grades so you can be the top of your class to create the most competitive medical school application. You work hard to differentiate yourself and demonstrate your uniqueness. In medical school, you work hard again to be at the top of your class, so you can be picked by the best residencies. Then, predictably, you're trying to be the best resident in order to be accepted at your chosen fellowship or land the best job. Then you go for a fellowship and guess what—you're trying to prove that you're the best fellow. This sequence does not naturally lend itself to the kind of training required for leadership.

For me, leadership entails something entirely different. It's about inspiring individuals to work together to achieve amazing results. It is about bringing ordinary people together to accomplish extraordinary things. The leader is not the one with the best ideas but rather the person that inspires others to come up with the best ideas, and choose the ones that are suitable for solving the problem at hand; to obtain agreement among team members and stakeholders, and to guide the team so that they obtain the desired results. In so many ways, I see leadership as the job of inspiring others to achieve, to fire them up and aim them at the problem to be solved. It requires an unselfish mindset that puts the team and project first. That's quite a different mindset from what we are taught in the traditional path of medical training.

Physician leadership can be taught and this teaching must encompass the entire career, starting with medical school and continuing through clinical training, and lifelong professional education after formal training is completed.

How does physician leadership impact work performance?

For us at USF Health, many of us were inspired by our former Dean Dr. Klasko, who presided over the creation of USF Health. His objective was to create a collaborative approach to healthcare, which led to the integration of the University of South Florida Morsani College of Medicine, the College of Nursing, the College of

Public Health, the College of Pharmacy, the School of Biomedical Sciences, the School of Physical Therapy and Rehabilitation Sciences, and the Doctors of USF Health. For him, physician leadership was a prerequisite for this integration and collaboration. The Physician Leadership Institute (PLI) itself was a spin-off from this exercise in collaborative innovation.

I remember how we participated in a specific workshop with the Physician Leadership Institute in which we were challenged to find a solution to a problem. The team stood around in a circle and tried to accomplish the challenge, with modest success. No one was speaking up. It occurred to me that as individuals who are trained to be right, physicians face an element of risk in voicing ideas or opinions that may be wrong. This leads many to avoid speaking up unless they are 100 percent certain that they are right. But this is not the way that unbelievably amazing things get accomplished. Amazing things get accomplished when we start out with less than perfect ideas and progressively improve them to get to the results we want to achieve.

I realized then that the job of the leader is to "make it safe to speak up." I offered a few suggestions, which were not very good ones, but what I learned and witnessed was that the initial, modest ideas led others on the team to offer progressively higher quality ideas.

Soon, we were hearing ideas from everyone and the best solution came, unexpectedly, from the physician who was the quietest one in the room.

In my role, I have the privilege of watching our fellows grow their clinical capabilities, work collaboratively, cover for each other, produce amazing results, while building a team culture above and beyond what I have seen in training before. The team feels more like a family now and I have to say, our fellows are doing magnificently, succeeding beyond our wildest expectations. Healthcare employers are taking note as well. Our fellows are being considered for some of the most competitive employment opportunities. That makes me think that we are producing a quality product.

What would you tell someone who is skeptical of the idea of physician leadership?

I would ask them to experience it before passing judgment.

Has physician leadership helped you beyond the workplace?

Doctors do not want to fail at anything they do. In fact, we practice risk avoidance and have made it an art. This is good in some areas. In other areas, however, it leads to scarcity of innovation and keeps us boxed in and victimized by our current set of problems. Physician leadership training has taught me to use failure as a tool for improvement, which leads to future successes. If you're not failing, you're not creating opportunities for future successes.

Each specialty has a set of fundamental principles, an evolving knowledge base, and the leader needs to master these in order to be able to guide and inspire the team. I also believe that if you take care of the basics, the fundamentals, the rest takes care of itself. This first lesson of leadership is something I try to practice in all aspects of my life.

What else would you like to add?

As our industry is challenged to improve accountability and outcomes, physicians are going to need to drive the change. For example, most doctors (myself included) do not know the costs of the treatment plans that we offer our patients. Many of us are disconnected from the business side of activities. I think that this is unacceptable. We need to gain a better understanding of the costs of the services that we offer to our patients so that we can help to drive these costs down.

Also, because of the increasingly interdisciplinary nature of patient care, doctors will be required to become more collaborative team players, skilled at initiating and managing change. That can't and won't happen without physician leadership.

INTERVIEW WITH DR. JOE COOPER

Dr. Joseph Cooper is a practicing board-certified ophthalmologist and a member of the American College of Physician Executives. He has been a member of the medical staff of Marietta (OH) Memorial Hospital for more than 25 years and has held numerous medical staff positions including department chair, credentials chair and president of the medical staff. He has also served as a hospital board trustee and chaired the board quality council. For the past eight years, Dr. Cooper has consulted with various medical staff on governance, credentialing and peer review. Recently he has also begun working with the Physician Leadership Institute. He consults with hospitals and medical staffs across the country in the areas of medical staff organizational functions, governance and bylaws, peer review, credentialing and privileging, and leadership training. He is a physician leader who brings more than 25 years of experience in medical staff functions and affairs to his work with physicians, hospitals and healthcare organizations across the country.

How do you view physician leadership? Can physician leadership be taught?

Definitely. There are some people who are born with it, but most people probably aren't. Just like any skill, it has to be taught; otherwise most people I don't think would have it.

Have things changed in your day-to-day activities as a result of taking physician leadership from the Physician Leadership Institute?

Definitely. In medical school, the problem is that you're not exposed to any leadership whatsoever.

You're exposed to clinical activity. You pick up either good or bad habits from who teaches you. And a lot of them don't have leadership skills either. So it's kind of catch-as-catch-can.

Most people get into a position starting to assume leadership and really have no training, with no insight whatsoever because it's not something that we've been exposed to for all those years.

They don't have classes or courses about leadership or teamwork. Maybe that world is changing now, maybe some of that is going to occur now. I know medicine is becoming more of a team sport compared to twenty years ago, but still I don't think they get much leadership in their formal training. My son just graduated from med school and there certainly wasn't anything like that for him.

Most doctors aren't exposed to leadership tools like we were in The Physician Leadership Institute, unless they've also completed an MBA or an MMM program. I think for the average doctor these things are very new. The leadership training is very valuable in that once you get exposed to it, it changes the way you approach and work with others. You start using different styles of interaction depending on the type of person you're dealing with. This is not something we were taught before.

In calm moments, we're humans. But in emergencies, we do become more technical—trying to make the best decisions to save a patient. All doctors have to learn to balance their emotions and their clinical skills.

In your opinion, who should enroll in these physician leadership programs?

If the people at the top are the only ones trained, it doesn't work as well. What you need is a culture of leadership and responsibility. Anybody can benefit from leadership training because everyone is a leader at one point or another. You see the benefit in interactions with others.

Doctors are autonomous animals, we were taught to do things by ourselves, make decisions on the fly all the time as I said. But to be a team player and look for consensus that's sometimes an alien world for even some very good doctors. Of course, there are some doctors who may say something like, "I don't have the time for this," but sometimes those are the very folks that need this training the most.

What would you tell someone who is skeptical of the idea of physician leadership?

I would tell them that there are benefits beyond simply your job. The benefits extend to your practice, whether it's a group or individual practice, and your day-to-day interactions with everyone you come into contact with. The life skills we learn, we also use with our families and friends. It is a transformative process not just for the organization but for individuals as well.

Did you notice an impact on business performance after the leadership training?

Because ours was a diverse group, I think the biggest changes you would see are in the groups that work together in the same organization or practices. Also, in teams that work together on action projects. Because of the personal coaching, you create specific plans for interactions with specific people. This was very helpful for me personally. I would hope that even my son would take a class like this so he could benefit from it for his future career.

A Call to Action: 7 Questions for The Leader

If you are ready to apply the Rx for healthcare transformation, think about these seven questions. Your answers will help you see what is required.

LEADING WITH PURPOSE:

☐ Is there a sense of purpose that is shared by and inspires physicians at all levels?

☐ Have we aligned and engaged the physicians in the transformation through a shared purpose and exciting possibilities?

LEADING WITH STRATEGY:

☐ Do we have a clear transformation strategy?

☐ Do we recognize that physician leadership is a critical success factor to the success of our transformation?

LEADING SELF:

☐ Do we have the right people as role models at every level to make this happen?

LEADING PEOPLE:

☐ As an organization, have we created a culture that values physician leadership?

LEADING FOR RESULTS:

☐ Have we given our physicians the necessary skills and experience through a fellowship to be successful and respected physician leaders?

BONUS QUESTION:

☐ Are we having fun? Why or why not? (Note: This is not a trick question!)

A Call to Action: 7 Questions for The Physician

If you are ready to apply the Rx for healthcare transformation, think about these seven questions. Your answers will help you see what is required.

LEADING WITH PURPOSE:

☐ Are you anchored in your deep purpose that got you into medicine?

LEADING WITH STRATEGY:

☐ Are you embracing healthcare uncertainty with courage?
☐ Do we recognize that your engagement and leadership is crucial to transform healthcare?

LEADING SELF:

☐ Do you see yourself as a leader and accept the professional mandate to lead?
☐ Are you managing your energy and wellness to prevent burnout?

LEADING PEOPLE:

☐ Have you created a habit and a culture to engage the hearts of others around you?

LEADING FOR RESULTS:

☐ Have you acquired the necessary skills and experience to be successful and an impactful physician leader (A Leaderist)?

BONUS QUESTION:

☐ Are we having fun? Why or why not? (Note: This is not a trick question!)

CONTACT US

The Physician Leadership Institute
www.physicianleadership.org

References and Bibliography

Physician Turnover Rate Rises With Economy, Robert Lowes, Medscape Medical news, March 18, 2013

Can Hospitals Heal Anemic Physician Engagement? Rick Blizzard, The Gallup Organization, September 2005

Exploring The Dynamics Of Physician Engagement And Leadership For Health System Improvement: Prospects for Canadian Healthcare Systems, ed. Lori Anderson, Canadian Foundation for Healthcare Improvement, April 2013

Burned Out, Ulrich Kraft, *Scientific American Mind,* June/July 2006 p. 28-33

When Clinicians Lead, James Mountford and Caroline Webbin, McKinsey Quarterly, February 2009

An empirical study in decline of empathy in medical school, M.Hojat et al., Medical Education, 2004 Sep 38(9): 934-941

Expert Culture versus Collaborative Culture

Can Hospitals Heal Anemic Physician Engagement? Rick Blizzard, The Gallup Organization, September 2005.

Exploring The Dynamics Of Physician Engagement And Leadership For Health System Improvement: Prospects for Canadian Healthcare Systems, ed. Lori Anderson, Canadian Foundation for Healthcare Improvement, April 2013.

Burned Out, Ulrich Kraft, *Scientific American Mind,* June/July 2006 p. 28-33.

Burnout and Satisfaction With Work-Life Balance Among US Physicians Relative to the General US Population, Arch Intern Med/Vol 172 (No. 18), October 8, 2012.

Stephen M. Shortell et al., *"An empirical assessment of high-performing medical groups: Results from a national study,"* Medical Care Research and Review, 2005, Volume 62, Number 4, pp. 407–34.

Lawrence Casalino et al., *"External incentives, information technology, and organized processes to improve health care quality for patients with chronic diseases,"* Journal of the American Medical Association, 2003, Volume 289, Number 4, pp. 434–41.

Innovation In The Kaiser Permanente Colorado Region, Bill Marsh MD and David Price MD, The Permanente Journal, 2005 Fall, 9(4): 40-43.

Ken Kizer, *Transforming The VA*, Medsphere, 2013.

BE-KNOW-DO, Leadership The Army Way, Leader to Leader Institute, Jossey-Bass, 2004.

Management: Tasks, Responsibilities, Practices; Peter Drucker, p.61.

Managing Oneself, Peter Drucker, *Best of HBR,* 1999.

Why Should Anyone Be Led By You, Robert Goffee and Gareth Jones, *Harvard Business Review*, Sept –Oct, 2000.

The Art of War, Sun Tzu

Why leadership-development programs fail: Pierre Gurdjian, Thomas Halbeisen, and Kevin Lane, *McKinsey Quarterly,* January 2014

Mezirow, J. *Learning as Transformation: Critical Perspectives on a Theory in Progress.* San Francisco: Jossey Bass, 2000.

Magill RA. *Motor Learning and Control*: Concepts and Applications. 2007.

Veloski, JJ., et al., 2006, Systematic Review of the Literature on Assessment, Feedback, and Physician' Clinical Performance: BEME Guide No 7. *Medical Teacher* 28(2): 117-28.

Atwater L., et al., 2007, Multisource Feedback: Lessons Learned and Implications for Practice. *Human Resource Management* 46(2): 285-307.

Tham, K., 2007, 360 Feedback for Emergency Physicians in Singapore. *Emergency Medicine* 24: 574-75.

Sergeant, JK et al., 2007 Challenges in Multi Source Feedback: Intended and Unintended Outcomes, *Medical Education* 41: 583-91.

Author Biography

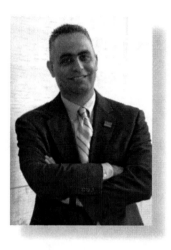

Mo (Mohamad) Kasti is the Chief Executive Officer and founder of the Physician Leadership Institute, specializing in empowering physicians to engage and lead the healthcare transformation.

An energetic and creative innovator with more than twenty-five years experience in healthcare and leadership, Mo has a keen ability to transform physicians, leaders and organizations. An award-winning and highly sought-after speaker, Mo trains and coaches physicians and leaders globally.

His passion and work to "change the DNA of medicine through leadership" have been praised by physicians, deans, hospital leaders and national organizations.

Mo has faculty appointments in the USF Colleges of Medicine, Nursing, Engineering, Business, and Pharmacy. He lives in Tampa, Florida with his wife and two sons. His blog is found at: www.mokasti.com, and he can be reached at: mkasti@physicianleadership.org

About the Physician Leadership Institute (PLI)

PLI uses evidence-based approach to empower physicians with necessary skills to lead positive healthcare transformation. Graduating physicians inspire their teams, collaborate with their peers and administrators, and deliver better clinical, service, and financial outcomes.

PLI offers a wide range of applied learning and formats that include:

- ☐ Assessment
- ☐ Physician coaching
- ☐ On-site workshops
- ☐ Strategy sessions
- ☐ Leadership academies
- ☐ Fellowships

For more information about the Physician Leadership Institute, visit: www.physicianleadership.org